Rethinking Prostitution

The growth of AIDS has focused renewed attention on the institution of prostitution. In contrast to the moral panic reaction of some sectors of society, very different initiatives are being displayed by other groups in relation to the need to scrutinize the social, moral and legal status of prostitution and to reflect on the arguments in support of or against legalising brothels, paying particular concern to prostitutes' own health.

Rethinking Prostitution covers male as well as female sex workers and considers in detail their status in law; drugs; issues of health and health care; the changing nature of sex work; partners, boyfriends and pimps; and the potential for redefining prostitution.

By drawing on the expertise of researchers across all aspects of the industry, this up-to-date text focuses on an institution and industry ripe for re-assessment. *Rethinking Prostitution* will be of considerable interest to students, lecturers and researchers in medical sociology and women's studies, social workers in training and practice as well as the general reader as an area of topical interest and concern.

Graham Scambler is Senior Lecturer in Sociology and Director of the Unit of Medical Sociology at University College London. **Annette Scambler** is an Honorary Lecturer in Sociology also at University College London.

Rethinking Prostitution

Purchasing Sex in the 1990s

Edited by Graham Scambler and
Annette Scambler

ROUTLEDGE

London and New York

First published 1997
by Routledge
11 New Fetter Lane, London EC4P 4EE

Simultaneously published in the USA and Canada
by Routledge
29 West 35th Street, New York, NY 10001

Typeset in Times by
Keystroke, Jacaranda Lodge, Wolverhampton

Printed and bound in Great Britain by
TJ Press (Padstow) Ltd, Padstow, Cornwall

British Library Cataloguing in Publication Data
A catalogue record for this book is available from the British Library

Library of Congress Cataloguing in Publication Data
Rethinking prostitution : purchasing sex in the 1990s / edited by
Graham Scambler and Annette Scambler
p. cm.
Includes bibliographical references and index.
1. Prostitution. 2. Sex oriented business. 3. Prostitutes–Social conditions. I. Scambler, Graham. II. Scambler, Annette, 1945– .
HQ117.R48 1997
306.74–dc20 96–21382
CIP

ISBN 0–415–12226–0 (hbk)
ISBN 0–415–10207–3 (pbk)

Contents

Part IV Health issues

Contributors

Niki Adams is a spokeswoman for the English Collective of Prostitutes. She is often on the media. She is widely consulted by working women, community and statutory organizations. She advised and was key to the first private prosecution for rape in England brought by two prostitute women after the Crown Prosecution Service dropped the case – the rapist was sentenced to 14 years imprisonment in 1995. She was central to the successful campaign to end the police and courts practice of using possession of condoms to arrest women for loitering and soliciting.

Peter Davis is Professor of Sociology and Health at the University of Portsmouth and Director of Sigma Research, an internationally renowned research group specializing in the study of sexual behaviour and HIV.

Sophie Day is a social anthropologist who holds appointments in the Department of Anthropology at Goldsmiths' College and the Department of Epidemiology and Public Health at Imperial College. She specializes in the anthropology of medicine, religion and sexuality, and has focused her work regionally in London and the Himalayas. She was the co-founder, with Helen Ward, of the Praed Street Project, an outreach and clinical service for prostitutes in London.

Susan Edwards BA, MA, PhD, LLM lectures in Law at the University of Buckingham. She has been writing and researching in the area of Sex and Gender and the Law for 20 years. She is actively involved in the work of several charities and voluntary organisations and has worked with the Coalition Against Trafficking in Women. Her latest book is *Sex and Gender in the Legal Process*, 1996, Blackstone Press, London

Dr Jean Faugier is Regional Director of Nursing at the NHS Executive North West. She trained as a psychiatric nurse and later as a psychotherapist. Prior to her current appointment she was senior lecturer at the University of Manchester Community Nursing Professional unit. She has undertaken a number of research projects investigating prostitution, HIV and drug misuse. The most recent of these was a study for the Department of Health about drug-using prostitutes and their risk behaviour.

Rayah Feldman is Principal Lecturer in Primary and Community Health Research at South Bank University, London. She has been involved in research on HIV/AIDS since 1991. Her recent work has been concerned with the provision of social care to families affected by HIV/AIDS. She is currently engaged in evaluating the impact of the East London childcare initiative. She has published work on women's health and on development issues in Africa with special reference to women.

Nina Lopez-Jones was part of the English Collective of Prostitutes Church Occupation in King's Cross in 1982. She researched and wrote the rights sheet 'Guide to the Rules of the Game for Working Girls' and is the editor of *Prostitute Women and AIDS: Resisting the Virus of Repression*. She is an internationally acknowledged expert on the prostitution laws and the co-ordinator of Legal Action for Women, the legal service initiated by the ECP.

Dr Maggie O'Neill is Senior Lecturer in Sociology and Women's Studies at Staffordshire University. She has worked for over six years conducting ethnographic research with women and young people working as prostitutes. This research is mostly collaborative participatory action research (with Prostitute Outreach Workers, Nottingham; the Stoke-on-Trent Sex Worker Project; and Rosemary Barbaret, University of Seville) which is committed to including the sterotypical subjects of research in the process and progress of the research. This involves working with and for women and young people involved in prostitution in a participation linked to the development of social research as social critique leading to changes in social policy and practice. Publications include work on the endemic nature of male violence against female prostitutes; the need for multi-agency approaches to prostitution which have prostitutes as key players; the need for multi-agency approaches to juvenile prostitution which revolve around the central role of the

Youth Service for the Children's Society; and the importance of feminist work on prostitution. *Prostitution and Feminism* is forthcoming with Polity Press in 1997.

Martin Plant PhD., a sociologist, is Professor of and Director of the Alcohol and Health Research Group. He has been engaged in research into alcohol, illicit drugs and other health and social issues since 1970. He is Professor and Director of the Alcohol and Health Research Group, Department of Psychiatry in the University of Edinburgh. During recent years his work has focused on alcohol control policies, teenage drinking habits, illicit drug use, sexual behaviour and risk-taking. His publications include the books *Drinking Careers*, *Drugs in Perspective*, *Risk Takers* and *AIDS, Drugs and Prostitution*. He is Meetings Secretary of the charity The Addictions Forum and is a consultant to the World Health Organization.

Mary Sargeant originally trained as a documentary photographer. She recently completed an MA in Applied Social Research at the University of Manchester and is now a research assistant in the Nursing Directorate at the NHS Executive North West. Her current research interests include mental health, women's issues, addictive behaviours and ethnographic research methods.

Annette Scambler teaches for the Open University and a number of London Medical Schools and is Honorary Lecturer in Sociology at University College London. Her main areas of interest are Women's Studies and gender issues in health care and the provision of care in the community. Recent publications include *Menstrual Disorders* (co-author 1993).

Graham Scambler is Senior Lecturer and Director of the Unit of Medical Sociology at University College London. His current areas of interest are the social theory of health and illness, chronic and stigmatizing conditions and the health of sex workers. Recent publications include *Menstrual Disorders* (co-author 1993), *Sociology as Applied to Medicine*, 4th edition (editor, forthcoming) and *Modernity, Medicine and Health* (co-editor, forthcoming).

Helen Ward is a Clinical Senior Lecturer in Epidemiology and Public Health at Imperial College School of Medicine in London. Since 1986 she has carried out research into HIV and sexual health in women working in prostitution. The research has led to the design and evaluation of interventions in various settings to reduce transmission of and morbidity from sexually transmitted infections. She was the co-founder, with Sophie Day, of the Praed Street Project, an outreach and clinical service for prostitutes in London.

Foreword

Understanding prostitution

Graham Scambler and Annette Scambler

INTRODUCTION

A cliché frequently used to introduce discussions of 'prostitution' claims it as one of the oldest of professions (e.g. Basserman 1967). Some caution is required however. 'Such "observations"', as Shrage (1989: 348) notes, 'take for granted that "prostitution" refers to a single trans-historical, transcultural activity'. The degree of continuity between the earliest documented forms of 'sacred prostitution' in the Middle East and contemporary Western 'secular prostitution' is in fact debatable. It is clear, for example, that in the cities of Mesopotamia and Egypt around 3000 BC, with the Great Goddess Innana (later Ishtar) herself identified as a 'prostitute', and with the 'prostitute-priestesses' of the temples still at the centre not only of religious but also political and economic power, 'the status of whores was high' (Roberts 1992: 4). In other words, these early 'prostitutes', as the *Epic of Gilgamesh* indicates, were far from being stigmatized as their putative counterparts in Britain are in the 1990s.

This volume is restricted to facets of prostitution, or the 'sex industry' (our preferred term), in Britain towards the end of the twentieth century. It is intended to inform and to stimulate discussion and debate, and perhaps also a 'rethinking', of sex work. In this Foreword we first note in passing some of the major theoretical perspectives on the sex industry and go on to outline some ideas of our own, and, second, explain the rationale for the contributions from colleagues that form the substance of the text.

SOCIAL THEORY AND THE SEX INDUSTRY

Over the years numerous sociologists and others have sought to develop or apply theoretical perspectives to the sex industry. The following categorization is far from exhaustive but illustrates something of the variety of theories in play and of levels of potential disagreement and dispute.

1 Sociobiological: these theories, sometimes characterized as Social Darwinist, start from the proposition that social difference, as found in sex roles for example, can be explained in terms of biological difference. Thus female prostitution or sex work is typically interpreted as a social imperative to accommodate the overpowering male sex drive.
2 Psycho- or socio-pathological: these theories seek the rationale for female sex work in some deep underlying pathology, be it in the (abnormal) psyches of women electing or willing to go on 'the game', or in the (abnormal) social milieux in which they were raised or interact.
3 Functional: these theories often betray biological origins, but they also insist that all social institutions through which sexual contact between men and women occurs are functional in some respect. Some maintain, for example, that female sex work is functional for marriage since it provides an outlet for excess – or deviant forms of – male sexual energy.
4 Conflictual: these theories emphasize female sex work's genesis in general social conflict of one type of another. According to some, for example, female sex work, is but a specific expression of the universal prostitution of the wage-labourer in capitalist societies. Women may be forced into sex work out of economic necessity, and 'forced labour' of this kind is the basis of social alienation.
5 Feminist: these theories typically draw on the concept of 'patriarchy'. In some, men's domination over women is seen as deriving from their control over female sexuality, manifest in social institutions like the family, heterosexuality and the female sex industry. Male control over female sexuality is underwritten by a patriarchal ideology which defines women as sexual objects, deprives them of their own sexuality and permits their violation by men.
6 Discourse analytic: these theories assert that the reading and practice of sexuality that underlie social institutions like the

female sex industry are not the conspiratorial product of powerful (male) agents; rather they are constituted in pre-eminent 'sexual discourses', which have their own histories and conditions of existence and are the truly appropriate objects of study.

While none of these six categories of theories is entirely convincing, and some in particular have lent themselves to ideological exploitation, each has something to offer. For example, it is possible to acknowledge the significance of biological differences between males and females without adopting a biologically determinist theory of the sex industry; it is possible to recognize that female sex work may help sustain pivotal institutions like marriage and the nuclear family without holding the view that all institutions can be understood in terms of their functions; and it is possible to assent to the proposition that women sex workers are often engaged in economically forced labour while denying that issues of class inequality have priority over or subsume issues of gender inequality.

It is not our purpose here to further explicate or provide critiques of specific theories of the sex industry (see Truong 1990). Nor is it our intention to profer an original theory or explanatory model of our own. Rather, it will suffice to elaborate on a few select – including some neglected – *themes* linking the British sex industry in the 1990s with what Giddens (1990) calls 'high modernity'. These are preceded by some general comments by way of a prolegomenon.

Historically, patriarchal relations, together with ideologies to legitimate them, preceded the advent of capitalism. Although British capitalism – from its early mercantilist to its later industrial stages – generated its own distinctive requirements, it did not in itself wholly determine the sexual identity of those obliged to fulfil these requirements. Capitalism in fact adapted to a pre-existing sexual division of labour in which men dominated women. Thus it was patriarchy rather than capitalism which prompted a gender-based differentiation of roles and tasks in the capitalist era. To accord historical priority to patriarchy here, however, is not to deny that capitalism went on to make its thoroughly distinctive mark on gender relations.

The predominant form of sexuality through this period has been aptly described as 'hierarchic heterosexuality' (Brittan 1989). Hierarchic heterosexuality is premised on an inequality of power between men and women: for example, men actively demand sex while women passively supply it. Hierarchic heterosexuality is not inevitable, it merely seems so because it has been taken for granted and reproduced in public and private spheres alike as if it were 'normal' and 'natural'.

Female sex work in Britain has to be understood against the background of the privileging of hierarchic heterosexuality in a capitalist economic system formed and consolidated in accordance with patriarchal relations. Moreover, it is in the work of women sex workers, some contend, that hierarchic heterosexuality is most publicly and explicitly revealed. For them, utilizing some key concepts of Habermas (1984, 1987; and see Scambler 1987), it is in female sex work that the (male) 'colonization' of sexuality via the 'steering media' of 'money' and 'power' can be most clearly discerned.

Money is the medium of the economic system, and women typically attract less for work outside the home than men, and many work for none inside the home. In the context of the pervasive ideology of hierarchic heterosexuality, it is men's access to money for the purchase of commodities in the capitalist marketplace, and women's lack of access to it, that underpins female sex work. And when men purchase sexual services from women sex workers for money, there is an important sense in which they transmute female sexuality into a commodity for men, one aspect of a much wider 'objectification' of women. The extent to which this echoes the routine experience of most women, sex worker and non-sex worker alike, remains a matter of controversy.

Power is the medium of the state. The political and state bureaucracy, through legislation and court and police activity, legitimates and reproduces hierarchic heterosexuality and, of course, regulates the sexual marketplace. The main British laws addressing the sex industry, together with their mode of reinforcement, serve to punish women sex workers, most notably street workers, for supplying sexual services in response to a steady demand from male clients. Even the Sexual Offences Acts of 1956 and 1985, aimed at third-party controllers and exploiters, and clients respectively, rarely hit their targets and, in their effects, cause most problems for women sex workers themselves (Scambler *et al.* 1990). Historical and contemporary study of state power in Britain shows a series of laws, made and enforced almost exclusively by men, the 'manifest' (e.g. Street Offences Act) or 'latent' (e.g. Sexual Offences Acts) function of which is to constrain female sexuality in line with the wider cultural norms of hierarchic heterosexuality (Merton 1968).

Thus far these preliminary paragraphs suggest that female sex work epitomizes the use and abuse of women by men, a position adopted by many feminists. This, we believe, is a partial truth which requires qualification. Certainly nobody who has observed a homeless 15-year-old girl high on drugs touting for business on the streets or treated a woman sadistically beaten by a pimp or client can be in any way sanguine. But a distinction has to be drawn between female sex work per se, and female sex work in a society characterized by patriarchal institutions and ideologies and capitalist economic relations. Too often these are conflated. However counter-intuitive it may seem, the link between female sex work and the use and abuse of women by men is contingent rather than necessary.

The themes we wish to identify here are mixed. The first concerns agency. Opposing the tendency, implicit in many social theories of prostitution, to regard women sex workers as more or less passive victims of their backgrounds or circumstances, we would advocate a *presumption of wilful rationality*. This is neither to deny the salience of background or circumstance for recruitment to the sex industry nor to assert that all engagement in sex work is a function of free and informed choice. Rather, it is to insist that the 'starting point' for any analysis be the respectful attribution of agency.

The second theme has to do with social changes which, in the recent years of the Thatcher–Major regimes, have consolidated or even extended gender-related disadvantages associated with recruitment to the sex industry. Material hardship is the most important and obvious of these. At the beginning of Thatcher's period in office McLeod (1982) characterized sex work as an 'act of resistance in the face of poverty'. Relative poverty in general, and female relative poverty in particular, has increased since then, not least under the auspices of a de-standardization of labour sometimes commended as 'flexible specialization'. Claims about the 'feminization of poverty' remain controversial in some quarters (Morris 1994), but there is no doubt that the rapid increase in lone-parent families, nine out of ten of which are headed by a woman, lend them substance (Lister 1992). As Oppenheim (1990: 98) notes:

> Many single parents are forced to rely on benefit even though many would prefer to be in work because they are caught in the unemployment trap. Childcare facilities are few and far between and are often expensive. The part-time jobs on offer are often low paid. As a consequence, many single mothers have little choice but to stay on benefit for several years. As all the evidence shows, long-term reliance on benefit means hardship and very often debt.

The housing problems facing lone mothers are no less daunting (Muir and Ross 1993). Against this background the English Collective of Prostitutes' (1992) estimate that nearly three-quarters of women sex workers are lone mothers is revealing.

The common observation by women sex workers that business has been slack during the last decade, which many attribute to a fear of HIV/AIDS on the part of potential clients, may in fact be due to enhanced competition for trade as more women confronted by hardship enter the industry, some of their number 'driven or recruited to sex work for want of alternative means to subsist or provide as single parents' (Scambler *et al.* 1990).

But there are other social changes in high modernity which may prove to have rather different implications for the sex industry. Our third theme identifies just a few of these. The first body of change issued from the second-wave feminism of the 1960s. While it would be easy to exaggerate the extent and durability of changes 'won' by feminist interventions in this decade, it remains true that not only did women extend and act upon their normative and legal 'rights' – both of access to hitherto male-dominated social enclaves (e.g. the upper echelons of the labour market) and of exit from hitherto female-'dominated' social enclaves (e.g. the domestic household) – but much patriarchal mythology was debunked in the process. New challenges to long taken-for-granted patterns of behaviour and thought, many reflecting a gendered 'double-standard' now readily castigated as intolerable, became commonplace.

A feature of this period too, and the second change we want to highlight, was the so-called 'sexual revolution'. Giddens (1992) has argued that this would have been unthinkable without the creation of what he calls 'plastic sexuality'. This refers to sexuality unharnessed from any intrinsic relation to reproduction. Together with plastic sexuality, of course, phenomena like the availability of contraception and divorce should also be noted.

The emergence of plastic sexuality might be profitably linked to a third change, namely, in the nature of relationships, including marital relationships. Beck and Beck-Gernsheim (1995) have argued that one property of high modernity has been an extended process of individualization. They identify three general phases: in the first, the family was essentially an economic unit, with neither partner possessing an individual biography; in the second, men were expected to take the initiative in organizing their own lives, family cohesion remaining intact at the expense of women's rights; and in the third, roughly since the 1960s, both men and women have been faced 'with the blessings and burdens of making a life of their own' (Beck and Beck-Gernsheim 1995: 76).

This third phase of the process of individualization has been characterized above all by the advent of the individual *female* biography. The authors (1995: 61–2) write:

> we are witnessing a new period in the history of women, and therefore in the history of men *and* women. Now for the first time two people falling in love find themselves both subject to the opportunities and hindrances of a biography designed by themselves.

High modernity, then, has featured not only a second wave of feminist advance and a sexual revolution predicated on plastic sexuality but a new kind of 'do-it-yourself-biography' (Berger *et al.* 1973). Beck and Beck-Gernsheim go on to maintain that this accent on individual biography, part and parcel of a de-traditionalized culture many designate as 'postmodern', militates against stable, monogamous, loving relationships (paradoxically, at a time when individuals are searching ever more anxiously for stability in precisely such relationships).

These themes around change are of course highly selective and our accounts of them overly succinct, but they do surely commend a reconsideration of the sex industry. After all, the role of women and the nature of sexuality and of relationships have all changed dramatically (one might perhaps add, even more than they have not changed, for it is always tempting to exaggerate change). Our hope is that this volume will both prompt some to a rethink of the sex industry, and prove a useful resource for others already committed or predisposed to just such a venture. It is intended as a contribution to an ongoing and increasingly vigorous, if often distorted, public debate.

The contributors were chosen for their expertise in the key areas of contemporary controversy and debate in Britain and were in each case invited to review the evidence and convey their own judgements. In Part I, Maggie O'Neill and Peter Davies give overviews of the social location and circumstances of female and male sex workers respectively. Part II starts with a review of prostitution law, with Susan Edwards emphasizing the need increasingly to consider the ramifications for the British sex industry of supra-national legal frameworks like that of the European Union. On behalf of the English Collective of Prostitutes (ECP), Niki Adams and Nina Lopez-Jones then give their own distinctive account of the parameters and utilization of British prostitution law and justify and document the ECP's campaign for reform. In Part III Graham Scambler focuses on the more neglected, mundane aspects of sex worker biographies, and Jean Faugier and Mary Sargeant draw on their own research to discuss crucial male participants in the sex industry, from clients to boyfriends and pimps. Part IV concerns health issues and drug use. Helen Ward and Sophie Day raise issues around the needs sex workers have for health care and problems of service delivery, their account informed by their work with the pioneering Praed Street Project at St Mary's Hospital, London. Martin Plant offers observations on drug use in the sex industry on the basis of a thorough review of his own and others' research. In the Afterword the editors reflect on some of the arguments for and against legalizing or decriminalizing sex work in Britain.

To borrow one of Habermas's phrases, if this volume assists the 'public use of reason' to reappraise the sex industry and the status and well-being of its workers it will have served its purpose.

Part I

An overview

Chapter 1

Prostitute women now

Maggie O'Neill

INTRODUCTION

In contemporary society prostitution, for some women, offers a good enough standard of income for shorter working hours and some degree of autonomy and independence for those working for themselves. Sex work has always been an alternative form of work for women (Henriques 1962; Finnegan 1979; Walkowitz 1980; Bullough and Bullough 1987; Day 1990; Meil Hobson 1990; Roberts 1992). But sex work also brings fear, violence, criminalization, stigmatization and reduced civil liberties and rights of human dignity, as well as the risk of disease and, for some, death.

The history of prostitution is one of immense contradictions as the prostitute is a figure represented in varying guises: whore/priestess, whore/goddess (Mesopotamia, circa second millennium BC). Whores achieved a certain level of autonomy leading to education and status within Ancient Greek society. They became bad girls, especially as the growth of Christianity and later Protestantism contrasted the ideal of the good wife and mother with bad girl and sinner. Increasingly within the Victorian period ideals of social purity and morality contrasted with dire economic poverty for working class/underclass women involved in a prolific sex-for-sale market, particularly in London (see Henriques 1962; Zola 1972: Finnegan 1979; Walkowitz 1980; Kishtainy 1982; Bullough and Bullough 1987; Roberts 1992).

Currently women working as prostitutes are perceived as bad girls, contravening norms of acceptable femininity, suffering whore stigma (Pheterson 1986) and increasingly criminalized by the state, policing practices and the lack of effective action taken by the state to address male violence against women (see Hanmer and

Saunders 1984; Hanmer and Maynard 1987; Hanmer *et al.* 1989; Hoigard and Finstaad 1992; Radford and Russell 1992; O'Neill 1993b, 1994, 1995). The social stigma and criminalization experienced by female prostitutes is further compounded by the masculinist organization and development of the sex-for-sale industry and the increasing feminization of poverty resulting in part from Conservative economic, employment and welfare policies in Britain, and the failure of social policies to fundamentally address the needs of the single female head of household.[1] Unequal sexual and social relations are ideologically and materially recip-rocal, underpinned and enacted by lived relations, by jurisprudence, by socioeconomic and cultural practices and processes.

The history of prostitution is a history framed by attempts to repress and make morally reprehensible the women involved in prostitution (Corbin 1987, 1990), whilst aestheticizing the desires and fantasies symbolically associated with the whore, the prostitute, the fallen woman. The history of prostitution is also tied to the history and social construction of sexuality, cathexis and the social organization of desire; gender relations; masculinity; and capitalist exchange relations which increasingly commodify everything, even love (Fromm 1967; Bertilson 1986; Luhmann 1986; Jackson 1993).

Some women working as prostitutes have spoken to me about the challenge prostitution poses to the nature of women's work in our society and to the representation of 'woman'.[2] Women's work is stereotypically associated with the ideology of domesticity and the private sphere, with long hours, little independence and/or autonomy. Representations and images of stereotypical femininity in contemporary culture are associated with the good wife and mother, the good girl, reliable, passive, nurturing, often fragile, gentle and emotional. Some whores claim to challenge these stereotypes for all women by resisting the pressure to conform to the stereotype of the good girl by bringing into the public sphere and to many men the services women usually perform in private for one man; and by insisting that prostitution is work, a service that anyone of age can offer or seek. For these women dressing as 'bad girls' reduces the power of patriarchy to divide women into madonnas and whores, thus destabilizing patriarchal power over women's bodies, sexualities, images and representations.[3] Furthermore, they claim that prostitution is work and that prostitutes should have the same rights and liberties as other workers.

By making the exchange relationship of money for sex (exchange value for use value) very public, by showing the heterosexual sexual encounter without the dressing of romance and romantic attachment, it could be argued that sex work and sex workers reveal inequalities within traditional heterosexual gender relations, particularly relating to 'masculinity(ies)' and the interrelated structures of work, sexuality and power (see Connell 1987) in contemporary society. 'All men make out that women's sexuality is dirty, but deep down it's their own they can't stand. So they blame women. We take it for all women, for all the others' (Jaget 1980: 93).

However, prostitution is double edged and any study of prostitution in contemporary society needs to face up to the contradictions inherent in the analysis and critique of prostitution whilst also offering support to women working as prostitutes (see Barry 1979; O'Neill 1994). For most women and young women working as prostitutes, economic need is the bottom line where entry into prostitution is concerned. Prostitution is accepted by bourgeois society (it is after all legal), but the whore or prostitute is not accepted. The prostitute is perceived as immoral, a danger, a threat to 'normal' femininity and, as a consequence, suffers social exclusion, marginalization and 'whore stigma'.

Sex, sin and morality: the politics of exclusion

Alain Corbin's (1990) analysis of commercial sex in nineteenth-century France describes how the interrelated discourses of municipal authorities, hygienists, the police and judiciary combined to organize the regulation of prostitution around three major issues: first, the need to protect public morality, articulated via concern to maintain the innocence of young girls 'from the spectacle of vice' (1990: 209); second, the need to protect male prosperity, for commercial sex was seen as a risk to social mobility and to patrimony; third, the need to protect the nation's health, for the prostitute was seen as an active agent for the transmission of disease. These three major issues are rooted for Corbin in five key images of the prostitute: first, the prostitute as the *putain* 'whose body smells bad' (1990: 210); second, the prostitute as the safety valve which 'enables the social body to excrete the excess of seminal fluid that causes her stench and rots her' (1990: 211); third, the prostitute as putrid body and sewer is symbolically associated with the corpse, with death (*Faculté* doctors used the corpses of prostitutes from the morgue for dissection purposes and hygenists' association of infection with rotting corpses, together with the symbolism associated with death and decay, further embedded the representation of the prostitute within sociocultural discourses of disease, decay and death); fourth, the symbolic association of the prostitute with syphilis; fifth, the prostitute as lower-class woman 'bound to the instinctive physical needs of upper class males' (1990: 213), submissive female bodies alongside the nurse, the nursery maid, 'the double faced servant, both Martha and Mary Magdalen, whose body serves as an object of obsession in the master's house' (1990: 213), and the old servant maid.

> Prostitutes, then, appeared dangerous for the same reason as corpses or carrion: . . . the ambiguous status of the woman's body, at once menace and remedy, agent of putrefication and drain . . . at the beck and call of the bourgeois body.
>
> (1990: 212–13)

Corbin goes on to illustrate how these discourses led to a series of principles which structured the regulation of prostitution. The principle of tolerances: as with all bodily functions we keep hidden but which are necessary for survival, prostitution is a necessary evil. The principle of containment: prostitutes should be isolated and contained away from purified public spaces. The principle of surveillance: contain and conceal, but keep under continual surveillance.

> The first task of regulation is to bring the prostitute out of the foul darkness and remove her from the clandestine swarming of vice, in order to drive her back into an enclosed space, under the purifying light of power.
>
> (1990: 215)

With the rise of utilitarianism the image of the brothel, 'a seminal drain' (1990: 215) closely supervised by the police, develops out of the image of the brothel, symbolic of debauchery, perversion, disease and decay.

The symbolic association of the prostitute/whore with death, decay, disease is maintained up to the present day.

> *Moira* I have lost friends, they look at you totally different . . . it bothered me. . . . I thought fucking hell I am a prostitute. . . .

> I am but I'm not. . . . I have two different lives . . . work and me . . . my boyfriend's friend sat watching telly and said 'Look at them dirty prostitutes' . . . and I said 'Just remember I am a prostitute and this is my settee paid for by prostitution and my TV and my carpet and everybody looked at me horrified'. . . . I was so horrified *in the beginning* . . . the first punter just wanted to look. . . . I had these durex and I wasn't even sure how to put it on properly. . . . I had real horrible nightmares that night . . . and I just counted my money, that was my comfort.
>
> (from a taped discussion with Jane, Sam, Moira, Susan and Mary 30 Sept. 1992, my italics)

Gail Pheterson's (1986) pioneering work in challenging the myths and symbolic associations of the prostitute with death, disease and decay is joined by the work of the Scamblers (1990), women themselves (Delacoste and Alexander 1988), and my own participatory action research with women working as prostitutes (O'Neill *et al.* 1995a, 1995b).

Prostitution now

What about prostitution today? Prostitution is not illegal, although in contemporary society it is perceived as a crime against morality. The prostitute stands outside mainstream society, is morally suspect and criminalized. Many women lead double lives to get over the problems associated with 'whore stigma'. Male violence against female prostitutes is endemic (Barry 1979, 1988; Hoigard and Finstad 1992; O'Neill 1992, 1993b, 1994, 1995). Women working on the street are constantly arrested for soliciting and suffer the extra burden of fines for their offence, followed for many by a stay in prison for fine default. Some women lose children to the care of the state (local authority) and sometimes do not manage to have their children returned to them if they are deemed 'unfit mothers'. The tragic irony here is that some women move into prostitution from the system of local authority care due to economic need, emotional neediness and vulnerability often related to peer pressure. Or they drift into prostitution within the context of a peer group whose members have in turn been let down by the system of local authority residential care.

Prostitution is a market for men; women are paid for the sexual services they perform on (with/for) men. Mary McIntosh has argued that issues of sexuality and sexual need are sociological rather than biological issues, and, further, that the 'ideology of male sexual needs both supports and is supported by the structures of male dominance, male privilege and monogamy' (1978: 3). Clients state that their involvement with prostitutes brings sex without commitment; thrills; compensation for a sterile marriage; sexual relief. Women experience relationships with clients some of which may be long-term friendships; others abusive and violent; others just business. Women who manage to 'make out' in prostitution talk about 'doing body work' and separating emotions from the physical embodied experience. Relationships with pimps are often business relationships, but can also be about 'love', 'dependency' and 'protection'. Much of the literature on prostitution focuses upon the women. We need to turn our attention to the men involved in prostitution. Masculinity(ies), problems within marriage and the family, and the aestheticization of the whore in contemporary culture (including media images and pornography) need to be explored to fully analyse and understand prostitution today (McLeod 1982; O'Neill 1993b).

What is clear to me is that women's lived experiences need to be contextualized within the gendered social, cultural, economic, historical and political backdrops to prostitution. The interrelationship between culturally situated lived experience and the wider social contexts need to be examined in order to develop policy-oriented practice to address the many issues and problems associated with prostitution, for all women. Socioeconomic structures mediate cultural practices. An exploration of the history of prostitution shows quite clearly that it is a cultural practice related to patriarchy. Walby (1989: 2) outlines how:

> the concept and theory of patriarchy is essential to capture the depth, pervasiveness and interconnectedness of different aspects of women's subordination, and can be developed in such a way to take account of the different forms of gender inequality over time, class and ethnic group.

Documenting the changing shape of patriarchy through time, Walby (1989: 24) argues we are living through a period of public patriarchy 'based principally in public sites such as employment and the state', and also through the patriarchal structures of household production, sexuality, violence and culture.

In everyday life our actions and choices take place within structures and practices already present and which are constantly being restructured by our very actions – the continuous structuring of structures (see Giddens 1984; Smith 1993). All our actions, intended and unintended, have the effect of structuring necessity, structuring gender, and gender relations (see Connell 1987). The law, the criminal justice system, social services, the health, welfare and benefit systems and the media are all instrumental in mediating prostitution as a cultural practice (and in turn are involved in the social reproduction and constitution of society). Knowledge about these agencies is central to understanding the circumstances, experiences and needs of prostitute women now. These major social agencies help to constrain and mediate the actions and attitudes of individuals by a mixture of service provision and the attitudes and behaviour towards prostitute women which they reinforce, legitimate or challenge.

My thesis here is that prostitution and the experiences of prostitute women now cannot be divorced from the socio-historical, cultural, economic and political contexts which mediate and give rise to prostitution in contemporary society. By exploring various kinds of empirical research and other academic text-based research in Britain and other countries, this chapter seeks to develop an overview of prostitution in the 1990s. Committed to a woman-centred analysis of prostitution and the development of feminist knowledge as feminist praxis (as knowledge 'for' see Stanley 1990), I will also seek to develop possibilities for relating contemporary research to practice-based work ongoing within the various agencies and institutions associated with prostitution. The intention is to relate theory to practice and practice to theory in a reflexive way geared to resisting, challenging and changing sexual and social inequalities for all women.

What follows is organized into two major sections. First, a description of what has changed and what has stayed the same since McLeod's ground-breaking work in the late 1970s and early 1980s, and the development of the major themes to be examined in the next section. Second, a section which follows on from McLeod and contextualizes these themes within a woman-centred overview and analysis of some of the current literature on prostitution now.

WOMEN WORKING

In 1982 Eileen McLeod published *Women Working: Prostitution Now*. McLeod, a feminist working with the Birmingham PROS

(Programme for Reform of the Law on Soliciting) street campaign in the late 1970s and early 1980s, was working with and for prostitute women. McLeod is concerned to show prostitutes as 'ordinary women', and, furthermore, that analysing prostitution may 'contribute to understanding more general social relations':

> as prostitutes, women are grappling with their disadvantaged social position in the context of a capitalist society. Recruitment to the ranks of prostitute is not appropriately characterised as only concerning a small group of highly deviant women. It is secured by women's relative poverty still being such that for large numbers sex is their most saleable commodity.
>
> (1982: 1)

For McLeod 'workers' control' is offset by male violence, male domination and superior purchasing power. The book relates the experiences of prostitute women, clients, the law/legal control and prostitutes' campaigns (community organization), concentrating largely on the street scene, and, together with Judith Walkowitz's *Prostitution in Victorian Society* (1980), was a great influence on my own work. Core themes in McLeod's book are working conditions, violence, male control, workers' control, disease, the law, prostitutes' campaigns and what clients want. McLeod examines street prostitution from a feminist perspective and incorporates the voices of female prostitutes and their clients.

Creating the intellectual and practical space for the voices of prostitute women is important in order to understand the lived experience of women working as prostitutes, but also to examine the resonances between their experiences and women's experiences more generally. Moreover, working with women in order to develop social knowledge as social critique is an important step on the road to a broader feminist emancipatory politics. But what exactly do we mean by prostitution and who are prostitute women?

Prostitution: what is it?

Prostitution is taken to mean the exchange of money for sex – use value for exchange value (as in all forms of work). Sex work is marked by the sale of sexual practices (intercourse, masturbation, S&M (sado-masochism), perhaps just a look at one's breasts) for money. For some, 'sex work' and 'sex worker' are preferred terms because they acknowledge the exchange of money for sex and are less stigmatizing than the terms 'prostitute' or 'whore'. Henriques (1962: 15) notes that the French definition of prostitution (which echoes the British legal definition) defines it as 'the partial or complete specialization of certain women in the satisfaction of the masculine instinct'. In the public imagination prostitution is a crime against morality; it is the women involved who are 'bad' girls, transgressing norms of femininity, culpable, even perhaps seen as dirty and disease-ridden. Yet, prostitution is a service for men. The demand for prostitution needs to be explored in relation to the commodity character of the sex industry and what Mary McIntosh (1978) has called the ideology of male sexual needs. More research needs to be done on masculinity, sexuality and the organization of desire in our society, linked to the regulation and surveillance associated with women in general and 'deviant' women in particular (see Smart 1992).

As far as prostitute women are concerned we need to move away from this idea that prostitute women are deviants or 'other'. Prostitute women, of course, are not all alike. As women we are multiple subjects situated by age, social class, race, sexual orientation and work. Our life experiences marked by our social situatedness have a great bearing upon the ways in which we see and give meaning to our lives and the wider social world. As women and multiple subjects, following Haraway (1991), we will inevitably develop different perspectives or ways of seeing at different points or stages in our lives. Speaking against the production of universal, totalizing theory which 'misses most of reality', Haraway emphasizes complexity, the creation and recreation of identities and categories indicative of the movement from industrial society to a 'polymorphous, information system'. My experience has shown me that prostitute women *are* ordinary women.

> *Sam* There is all different reasons why you go into prostitution. . . . I went into it through choice and if I decide to stop it might happen this year or next year . . . but I can't see it because I am not ready to. I have good clients and I am not prepared to give up them dollars for love or money . . . I have always known I have high self-esteem because I have other skills and I think; don't think every prostitute has low self-esteem because every prostitute hasn't . . . once you start stigmatizing prostitution,

> girls start having low self-esteem; once a woman starts believing in herself she can decide for herself . . . go back to college or work in the co-op . . . how many women prostitute themselves in relationships they don't want to be in but stay in a marriage for financial gain? If it wasn't for financial gain how many women would walk out of that relationship?
>
> (from a taped discussion with Sam, Jane, Moira, Susan and Mary, 30 Sept. 1992)

Materially, prostitution is often a response to poverty, financial hardship and need. We need to be aware of changes in the benefit system, changes in the care system, changes around the employment of young people, including YTS, the council tax, student grants, recession and high interest rates, which increase the risk of more people and more young people becoming involved in prostitution (see Lupton 1985; O'Mahoney, 1988; Newman 1989; Stein 1990; Dibblin 1991; O'Neill 1991; Walklate 1991; Biehal *et al.* 1992).

As a response to poverty, selling sex is often a last resort, the body one's last commodity. We cannot look at prostitution without looking at the social and economic contexts which give rise to it. The majority of women's work is part time, low status and low paid. There is an absence of good quality child care facilities. There is an increasing number of young people, disenfranchised, disaffected and homeless:

> women bear the burden of managing poverty on a day-to-day basis. Whether they live alone or with a partner, on benefits or low earnings, it is usually women who are responsible for making ends meet and for managing the debts which arise when they don't. Indeed, the lower the household income, the more likely it is that this responsibility will rest with women. As more women and men lose their jobs, and as benefits are cut or decline in value, women are increasingly caught in a daily struggle to feed and clothe their families – usually only at considerable personal sacrifice.
>
> (Glendinning 1987: 60)

Morally and ideologically the implications and responses to sex work are historically rooted in a double standard of morality reflected in the laws around soliciting and kerb-crawling, as well as embedded in the whole process of socialization (see Lees 1993). Pheterson (1986: 227) writes with feeling about what she calls the social consequences of unchastity and the shaming of young girls, i.e., 'unchastity' as an excuse for 'male sexual violation'. But, more than this, in equating whore status to unchastity, unchastity can be used to 'justify oppression and abuse'. Furthermore, 'any woman is vulnerable to the whore stigma as a result of life experience, sexist abuse, or ill fortune'.

Prostitutes: who are they?

Who are prostitutes? They are women, men and young people who come from all social classes, although the majority of women working as prostitutes tend not to come from the middle classes. McLeod (1982: 26–7) documents becoming a prostitute as a way out of relative poverty through the accounts of Rosa, Carol, Julie and Kathy. She stresses also personal biography 'in connection with local conditions, such as the existence of a number of women working as prostitutes and more structural forces such as employment opportunities' (1982: 33–4). She suggests too that an independent cast of mind and a degree of isolation or distance from one's family, including emotional distancing, are instrumental for some women. This picture is reflected in the literature. Teachers and nurses have been documented as moving in to prostitution (escort and working from home), tired of earning so little for the social services they perform (*New Statesman and Society* 1990), as have executives supplementing salaries and supporting increased mortgage payments through escort work (*Company* 1990: 42–3), students (Delacoste and Alexander 1988; *Sunday Correspondent* 1990; *Video Diaries*, BBC 2 September 1993), women supplementing social security payments or low incomes (Jaget 1980; Edwards 1988a, 1988b; O'Neill 1994, 1995) and women with no formal skills or training, or no confidence, sense of self-worth or self-esteem (O'Neill 1995). Often the latter group have a history of homelessness, poverty and loneliness. Some women feel they may as well be paid for doing what they are expected to do for free.[4]

Women and young people are sometimes coerced into prostitution through relationships with men and sometimes women. I met Sarah in September of 1992. She was 14 years old and had become involved in prostitution through her friendship with other girls. In and out of care from the age of eight Sarah worked for money for 'draw' and cigarettes; she used to work for money for 'crack'. She didn't go to school because she 'didn't fit in'. With professional help she came off crack but was still working, particularly when she was bored. Sarah had been slashed, beaten and raped in the course of her work as a prostitute (O'Neill 1995).

Young people can become involved in prostitution through emotional neediness and vulnerability as well as homelessness and poverty. In my work with and for women and young women I have met young people ill-equipped for independent living who have had little continuity of care, being moved from foster care to residential care or between residential homes numerous times. Losing out on education, in part due to the culture of care, low self-confidence and self-esteem, they cling to a peer group offering a sense of belonging and mutual support.

> *Beth* At the beginning I remember being in care and I can remember a girl who used to work; I used to go out with her and wait for her and I can remember it was a tiny little community and prostitution wasn't as big as it is now. I wanted to belong, it had got nothing to do with money. I went in as a mixed up little kid.
>
> *Maggie* So you went in from care?
>
> *Beth* Yes, well I used to sneak out the windows at night . . . but it was just I followed the flow. . . . I didn't make any decisions.
>
> (From a life-history interview with Beth, Sept. 1992)

Some of these are individuals with a history of abuse. One young woman began to work as a prostitute from a community home when she became involved in prostitution through her friendship with another girl who worked. She 'just went along' with her friend and had been working eighteen months when I met her. Her entry at 14 into local authority care followed sexual abuse from her step father. She began to work as a prostitute at 16. A young man who had suffered a sexual assault told me how he compulsively returned to the scene of the assault and began working as a prostitute until he was able to unburden himself to a social worker, who was then able to help him begin to recover his self-esteem, confidence and ability to distinguish his own sexual needs from self-harm by organizing counselling and giving him care and support. Some young people I have talked to began working as prostitutes on leaving local authority care due to problems related to economic need and lack of employment.

Routes in to prostitution

Routes in to prostitution are varied. Some women make independent lifestyle choices due to the realities of economic need in a climate of economic recession, inadequate benefits, unemployment and increasing debt. Women sometimes drift in through association with friends already working. An option not thought of before presents itself and a decision to try prostitution is made. Young women drift in to prostitution through peer association and peer pressure. Coercion from pimps is not uncommon. Prostitution in order to make the money to support one's own or another's drug habit is not uncommon. The links between local authority care and drifting into prostitution need to be thoroughly researched in order to develop intervention strategies around prevention and minimization of harm. Specifically, the relationship between prostitution and residential care has to be explored within the context of the experiences and problems which bring young people into the care of the local authority; the residential care experience itself and the social stigma, marginalization and 'otherness' related to being in care; financial resources allocated, training and education of social workers and carers; the overall management of care; the benefit system for young people; education, employment and training opportunities. There is little point in blaming social services or the system of residential local authority care for young people's involvement or drift in to prostitution. What we ought to be doing in policy terms is ensuring that the system of residential care is adequately funded, staffed and resourced to meet the needs of needy children and young people who are sometimes very damaged by their life experiences (O'Neill *et al.* 1995a).

Socioeconomic, cultural and political contexts to prostituting now

What we must be clear about is the socioeconomic context to prostitution, which includes: the activities of the state; the activities of those institutions and agencies (statutory and voluntary) working with and for prostitute women; inequalities of income, education, welfare and health, employment and training opportunities; the realities of sexual and social oppression; the increasing feminization of poverty; male violence, gender relations – masculinity and the social organization of desire. Above all we need to avoid maintaining and reproducing the ideology of prostitution. By the ideological

I mean that which serves to conceal unequal and oppressive sexual and social relations and practices. Sectional interests presented as universal interests, the denial of contradictions and the naturalization of that which has been socially constructed are all examples of ideological effects (Giddens 1984).

There have been many social changes since McLeod's book was written. A further fourteen years of Conservative government in Britain and of global economic recession have brought a great increase in the feminization of poverty; an increase in young women and men working as prostitutes often in exchange for a bed or food; an increase in those working in the sex industry as prostitutes, strippers, erotic dancers, hostesses due to the realities of economic need. We have witnessed an increase in forced and voluntary prostitution in Third World countries, sexual tourism and trafficking. There has been a growth of prostitutes' rights campaigns and grassroots organizations working with prostitutes. More recently there has been an increase in academic research and information on prostitution, much of this funded by public health monies.

In Britain some local authorities are in the process of creating, or have considered creating, zones of tolerance where prostitution can take place (Ryle 1992). Currently an all-party parliamentary group on prostitution is meeting to explore the way forward with particular reference to law reform. Women working as prostitutes, health and welfare agencies, and the police have been invited to give evidence. Prostitution is no longer an imprisonable offence, although women do get sentenced to prison for fine default. The clients of prostitutes are now criminalized through the 1985 Street Offences Act for the offence of kerb-crawling. There has also been an increase in male prostitution and transsexual prostitution.

The global AIDS pandemic has changed the face of sexual encounters and sexual practices, and in the Western world initially prostitutes were blamed for the transmission of the virus into the heterosexual population. Empirical evidence gathered from a number of UK studies (for Praed Street Project in London see *Forum* 1989; for the Safe Project in Birmingham see Kinnell 1989, 1991; in Glasgow McKeganey and Barnard, 1992a, 1992b) and international studies (Leukefeld *et al.* 1990) have shown categorically that women working as prostitutes are fastidious in their use of condoms. Peer education programmes (such as SCOT-PEP and POW!) have shown that prostitutes are excellent peer educators on safe sex practice. However, their clients are not so conscious of the risks. Many men ask and pay more for sex without the use of condoms. Given the profile of the average punter this evidence is very worrying and has implications for the transmis-sion of HIV to their regular partners as well as alerting health educators to the need for better campaigns aimed at the heterosexual population.

Some things have changed very little since McLeod's book was written. Male violence against women remains endemic. Street prostitution in Britain is still largely controlled by men acting as pimps/ponces. The financial organization and control of the wider sex industry (including pornography) remains in the hands of men. Women are still criminalized and stigmatized for their activities. It is still very difficult to work as a prostitute and remain within the law. 'Common prostitute' is still the label given to women following two cautions. Women are still carrying huge fines, being sent to prison for fine default, losing children to local authority care, and sometimes their partners are imprisoned for the offence of living off immoral earnings. The high-profile policing of prostitutes continues to increase the risks to women particularly relating to their personal safety.

The following section takes a closer look at the wider international context to prostitution and some of the literature and empirical research from a woman-centred perspective.

A WOMAN-CENTERED ANALYSIS OF THE WIDER SOCIO-POLITICAL CONTEXT: CONTINUITY AND CHANGE

The feminization of poverty, global recession, problems in marriage and the family within the context of changing demographic structures and the freeing up (de-traditionalization) of large aspects of social life (see Haraway 1991; Beck 1992; Giddens 1992; Haug 1992), unequal sexual relations, lack of action by the state to fundamentally deal with increasing poverty for women and children and the endemic nature of male violence against women (Hanmer and Maynard 1987; Kelly 1988; Hanmer *et al.* 1989; Radford and Russell 1992), the ideology of 'whore stigma' and a criminal justice system which prosecutes prostitutes on the basis of outmoded legislation all combine to shape the causes and context of female prostitution now.

Internationally there have been some changes in the social organization of prostitution. Evidence from France (Welzer-Lang, 1993) suggests that prostitution is undergoing changes in its organization and structures. Welzer-Lang's research in progress has documented a reduction in the numbers of visible female prostitutes on the street, an increase in male prostitution (one in three are men), an increase in transsexuals working as prostitutes, increasing self-organization and regulation of prostitution by women themselves, and new forms of sexual services, e.g. machine sexuality (telephone sex), coinciding with the AIDS era.

The social organization of prostitution has undoubtedly been affected by the growing voice and influence of the 'prostitutes' rights' movement, the links with feminism and the rise of grassroots organizations supported by 'experts' and 'professionals'. Furthermore, the increase in sexual tourism, the feminization of poverty, the development and management of the sex trade in Third World countries, AIDS, and the problems associated with political and economic change in Eastern Europe all influence the social organization of prostitution on a global as well as a national level. These changes or shifts need to be explored within the context of social processes, social order and social change more generally. They also need to be accounted for and explored through empirical research, taking an ethnographic approach, and contextualized within comparative historical research. Europeanization, transnational research links, and the sharing of information, knowledge, methods and methodologies have a bearing and influence upon the agencies working with and for prostitute women, attitudes to prostitute women, and the ways in which the prostitute enters the public imagination. Such links also have a part to play in developing policy-oriented practice around the issues and problems associated with prostitution. Education and training programmes supported by prostitutes, for prostitutes, ex-prostitutes and daughters of prostitutes are one example. APRAMP operates from Madrid: a team of social workers, educationalists, counsellors and prostitute outreach workers deliver and organize services for prostitutes of all ages and their daughters.[5] APRAMP offer apartments for women, temporarily or on a longer-term basis; outreach services; a programme which includes counselling and therapeutic services, education and training; help with legal, welfare and social needs.

An overview of some of the contemporary literature

Critical analysis of the available literature problematizes some of the issues raised here. Questions to do with the routes women take into prostitution, of what happens to women in terms of material, practical, and emotional support and resources whilst engaged in sex work, in 'making out', and also how women might leave sex work if they want to, cannot be answered unless the literature is analysed from a woman-centred perspective. A woman-centred perspective must engage with the socioeconomic and political contexts of women's involvement in sex work, and the moral and ideological approaches to sex work and sex workers which form the backdrop and indeed underpin the experience of being a prostitute in contemporary society.

Historical analysis (Henriques 1962; Walkowitz 1980; Kishtainy 1982; Corbin 1990; Roberts 1992) points to the relationships between whores, the state, working-class communities and the regulation of the body, knowledge of the role and position of women in society, and the fact that prostitution has always been work that women can engage in in order to make a living. Historical analysis can also, as Corbin shows us, reveal the trends and shifts in moral, ideological and symbolic images and associations relating to prostitution and the prostitute.

Sociological and criminological work in the area has been relatively sparse. Mary McIntosh (1978), Eileen McLeod (1982) and Susan Edwards (1988a, 1988b), writing from feminist perspectives, highlight the problematic relationships with clients (male needs), the law and policing practices. They also stress the economic reality for many women which underpins their entry into prostitution. Issues of sexual politics are entwined with economic and political issues – housing, benefits, health, welfare and the feminization of poverty combine to create a catch-22 situation for women who may not have freely chosen to work as prostitutes but nevertheless pragmatically have decided that this is the best option available to them.

Suzy Kruhse-Mountburton (1992: 225) evaluates the Australian legislation on prostitution and concludes that decriminalization is the only rational strategy 'in a community which affirms a policy of advancing the status of women, while the legal system condemns some of their number for a sexual behaviour fashioned to please men'. Moreover, quoting Barton *et al.* (1987):

> Public health measures should be directed at the clients of prostitutes to increase their appreciation of the protection afforded by condom use and the need for regular medical examinations to detect asymptomatic infections . . .
>
> (1992: 226)

Kruhse-Mountburton stresses that the rate of infection of HIV tends to be low or absent in non-drug-using prostitutes, but that clients are the 'largest component of the prostitution industry . . . their attitudes and behaviour . . . largely determines the impact of prostitution on the community in terms of S.T.Ds' (1992: 224). Furthermore, 80 per cent of the male population might be expected to interact with a prostitute at least once. Kinsey (1948) gives a figure of 69 per cent of the adult male population, while for Benjamin and Masters (1965) 80 per cent is a more realistic figure. Kruhse-Mountburton is against regulationism; for her, decriminalization with safeguards would 'eliminate the need for prostitutes to walk the precarious legal tightrope presented to them by the current legislation' (1992: 221).

Policing initiatives coming from anti-vice squads and sometimes drug squads point to the problems for residents living in areas where women work on the street and the need for policing to respond to residents' needs, as street crimes, soliciting and kerb-crawling create nuisance for residents. Golding (1992) has written about the lack of national standards in the policing of prostitution. Fines vary in accordance with magistrates' interpretations of the system. In my own area, the anti-vice squad has a three-pronged approach to prostitution. Women are arrested for soliciting, charged and usually fined. Punters (clients) are fined for the offence of kerb-crawling at a rate of £100 plus court costs. Those men who are persistent drivers in the area are bound over to keep the peace for one year. Pimps (coercive men not usually partners or grown-up children), once arrested and charged, have to prove they are not living off immoral earnings. Police prove association by gathering evidence from surveillance activities.

Roger Matthews (1986, 1991), writing in England from a socialist, left-realist position, has explored the legacy of Wolfenden (1957) and the problems inherent in legalizing prostitution in contemporary Britain. For Matthews, multi-agency approaches to street prostitution, including road closures and traffic calming measures, benefit residents and also help to deter or deflect some women from street prostitution. Matthews also examines the legalization/decriminalization debate, and the socio-legal context to prostitution and the law, and suggests an approach he calls 'radical regulationism' to deal with the issues and problems prostitution raises. Radical regulationism speaks of 'protective intervention' and is based upon a model which stands firmly on the side of residents in 'red-light areas' in partnership with the police and the city or borough council.

Matthews' multi-agency approach does not allow for women working as prostitutes to become involved in discussions or decision-making. Multi-agency approaches to prostitution which are 'women centred' can allow for a more coordinated network of services to prostitutes, playing educative and empowering roles, as well as fostering greater inter-agency cooperation and communication so long as prostitute women are key players (O'Neill 1991, 1993a). Multi-agency initiatives informed by wider social, legal and economic processes as well as a better understanding of the lived experience and needs of women working as prostitutes can move forward in more informed ways. The multi-agency approaches operating in the East Midlands and West Midlands are vastly different from those operating in Luton, Southampton and Streatham. The latter are about law enforcement agencies and county councils getting together to develop a system of higher fines, high-profile policing, road closures and traffic management schemes, which serve only to displace the 'problem' and do not consider the women involved, their needs, rights or status as 'normal women'. Multi-agency approaches, working together with prostitutes' rights groups, could develop recommendations aimed at policy change which reflect the lived experience of prostitute women, their material/economic as well as health, welfare and emotional needs. Feminists involved in such multi-agency groups need to face up to the contradictions inherent in working with and for prostitute women whilst finding the institution(alization) of prostitution problematic (see also Barry 1979, 1988).

John Lowman (1992a, 1992b), who is critical of Matthews, has explored the situation in Canada over a number of years and develops the legalization/decriminalization debate by addressing the changing geography of street prostitution in relation to law enforcement, and suggests a legal system which identifies where prostitutes can work and which protects women from violence. Critical of both the government and 'the contradictory and self-defeating nature of the various Criminal Code sections', Lowman also focuses upon the need to address the purchasers of women's services, patriarchal social relations, age and gender employment structures, and the feminization of poverty.

Johannes Boutellier (1991) develops the legalization/decriminalization debate from the perspective of prostitution, criminal law and morality in the Netherlands, and interestingly hangs this upon the involvement of leading feminists. A coalition between feminists and local government agencies has changed the public debate on prostitution. In 1985 the government changed the article on brothel-keeping (250bis) which had been instantiated in the 1911 Public Morality Act. 'Brothel-keeping was no longer to be prohibited, except for cases of violence, force or overpowering (1991: 201). The revision of the law facilitates prostitution being perceived as work, but there is concern about the relationship between prostitution as work and prostitution as traffic in women. Currently feminists in the Netherlands are clear about their stance. Prostitute women should not be blamed; instead the men who organize them and visit them should hold responsibility. Judicial policy should look towards brothel-keepers *not* the women who work there. Improving the socio-legal standing of women is central to the feminist cause. Boutellier documents the shifts in feminist approaches to prostitution, from the coalition with the social purists in the early part of this century, to the emphasis upon prostitution as a psycho-social problem and the need for rehabilitation to reinforce family ties and male moral standards in the post-war years, to the current situation which Boutellier calls 'moral indifference'. The late 1960s and 1970s are seen as times of sexual liberation. The Melai Committee in 1977 warned the government against intruding into the private sphere and pleaded for selective action against exploitation of individuals and nuisance to residents/neighbours. The debate was one which focused upon the management and control of prostitution. Prostitution is a 'technical-juridical problem of public order' (1991: 206). Sixteen years later, the debate over the legalization (regulation) or decriminalization of prostitution is now being waged in Britain.

For Boutellier there are two major feminist approaches. The first views prostitutes as victims of male sexuality: thus male sexuality should be the main subject of concern' (1991: 207). The second 'subjectivist' position places the experiences and needs of the women concerned centre stage and views prostitution 'as a legitimate form of labour freely chosen by thousands of women' (1991: 207). Government policy is unnecessary once proper conditions for this work are established. For Boutellier, this approach is compatible with the 'morally indifferent technocratic approach absorbed with management and control'. Boutellier ascribes this shift in part to social changes in what is termed 'moral judgement':

> Until the 1960's moral judgements were part of the encompassing political ideologies of a religious socialist or liberal kind. Lately, these ideologies – at least in the Netherlands – seem to have lost their importance in defining social problems. This change is often referred to as the 'individualisation' of society. . . . Morality today might more usefully be seen as the mediation between individual experience and state bureaucracy. . . . The prostitution issue is not nearly what it once so much was – an issue of ideologically defined morality – but an issue about the subjective experiences of the persons involved and the bureaucratic necessity of regulations.
>
> (1991: 209)

It is too simple to reduce the feminist approaches to prostitution to these two diametrically opposed perspectives; the situation is much more complex and contradictory. The European and international prostitutes' rights organizations are calling for prostitution to be seen and taken as work, asserting that women should have the same rights and liberties as other workers. Many whores who are also feminists or feminist-informed are arguing that the realities of women's lives do not necessarily give them the opportunity to engage in a debate about male oppression and the problems related to supporting patriarchy (McLintock 1992). However, many women involved in these organizations, and women working as prostitutes, are aware of and antagonistic to the involvement of men as pimps, ponces and abusers of women working as prostitutes. Strategies of resistance are developed and shared between women around self-help, support and peer group empowerment/education.

On the other hand, as argued most notably by Kathleen Barry, we cannot turn a blind eye to the horror of international trafficking in women and children when exploring possibilities, both practical and ideological, for sanctioning the use value for exchange value of women's bodies, or prostitution as work. Furthermore, as Carole Pateman argued in 1983:

> Neither contempt for women nor their ancient profession underlies feminist arguments; rather, they are sad and angry about what the demand for prostitution reveals of the general character of (private and public) relations between the sexes. The claim that what is really wrong with prostitution is hypocrisy and outdated attitudes to sex is the tribute that liberal permissiveness pays to political mystification.
>
> (1983: 565)

For Pateman, prostitution needs to be 'placed in the social context of the structure of sexual relations between men and women' (1983: 563). My own work has looked at prostitution from a feminist 'woman-centred' position. In it I acknowledge the lived experiences of women working as prostitutes within the context of sexual and social inequalities and aim to give sex workers a voice by working with them through participatory action research. A key aspect is the reflexive interrelationship between feminist theory, women's lived experience and policy-oriented practice articulated through feminist participatory action research. Prostitution and violence, prostitution and the state, feminism, prostitution and the political economy, and the social organization of prostitution (at a national as well as a European level), the management of female sexuality, sexual trafficking and tourism, are central themes and concerns.

Feminist analyses of prostitution inevitably challenge the ways in which sexual and social inequalities serve to reproduce ideology, patriarchy and the structuration of gender relations. The central ideological problem for feminism is that the exchange of money for sex is taken to be the exchange of equivalents. This is a socially created illusion and is central to the commodification of women's bodies as use objects and our subsequent oppression in society. Both first- and second-wave feminists have fought battles based on the use value of women and women's bodies. However, feminism must acknowledge that, for some women, prostitution gives a good enough standard of income and relative autonomy, and can be fitted in around child care. Focusing upon the moral rights and wrongs of prostitution and the enforcement of a justice model based upon Victorian ideology and Wolfenden (which criminalizes and stigmatizes the whore but not her client) hides the gender issues implicated in the question: why do men use prostitutes? It is this issue which needs to be given more attention whilst at the same time working with prostitutes' rights organizations to address sexual and social inequalities.

Feminism and feminists must face up to the contradictions inherent in working with and for prostitute women and call for the return of civil liberties and rights of human dignity to prostitutes; they must also call for direct action from all those agencies working with prostitutes, particularly at the level of the criminal justice system, to explore their policies, codes of practice and funding mechanisms in order to enable working women to be given a better deal. Feminists necessarily challenge the discrimination and oppression of women; whores are women first and support for women's rights should not be divided. Creating a space for women involved in prostitution to be heard, and in turn for feminist research to inform theory and practice around women's involvement in the sex industry, is at the very heart of my own approach.

We need to explore the social organization of prostitution in all its complexity. This includes looking at the agencies working with and for prostitute women, which necessarily affect and are affected by the experiences of women working as prostitutes. Contextualizing our knowledge within a broad understanding of prostitution, the social order and social change in contemporary times, we may be able to move towards recommending changes in social policy and developing concerted action to help effect change.

Women-centred research informing both theory and practice

Research on health issues for prostitute women points to the problematic nature of the interest in prostitute women's health (see Scambler and Scambler 1992). Scapegoated for transmission of AIDS to the general population through unprotected contacts with clients, perceived as health educators of their client group, eventually prostitutes were perceived as recipients of health care and protection in their own right. Health-based research and practice has been instrumental in supporting and developing some pioneering work in Britain. The Safe Project in Birmingham; the Praed Street Project based at St Mary's Hospital in Paddington; SCOT-PEP and the Centenary Project in Edinburgh; the Health Shop and POW! (Prostitute Outreach Workers) based in Nottingham; WHIP (Women's Health in Prostitution Project) in Leicester; the Wandsworth Female Sex Workers Project; the Cardiff Outreach Project and the Sheffield AIDS Education Project are but a few examples. POW! in Nottingham, WHIP in Leicester and Soliciting for Change in Caldmore, Birmingham are the three I am most familiar with.[6]

Information, education and support around women's self-empowerment are aspects of the work undertaken at the projects named above. Data collected particularly from the Safe Project (Kinnell 1989, 1991) and the Praed St Project (*Forum* 1989) as well as from McKeganey and his colleagues in Glasgow (McKeganey 1992; McKeganey and Barnard 1992a, 1992b; McKeganey *et al.* 1990, 1992), Morgan-Thomas *et al.* in Edinburgh (1989, 1990), Plant (1990) and Green (1992) have developed greater awareness and understanding of working women's health and welfare needs and circumstances. Such data were instrumental in de-bunking the idea in the public imagination of the dirty, disease-ridden prostitute. It became clear that women working as prostitutes are very conscious of their health needs and are taking precautions against the risk of contracting STDs, including AIDS. Health agencies particularly have been instrumental in developing research which generates better information about the extent of prostitution and the male client group, but which also develops services to support and empower prostitute women.

Prostitutes' rights and grassroots organizations are an important development of recent years; probably *the* most important development. SCOT-PEP and the Centenary Project can be counted among such organizations. In the last two to three years there has also been a noticeable development of grassroots organizations.

Valerie Jennes (1990, 1993) shifts the debate about prostitution away from discourse about sin, sex and crime, placing it within a discourse about work, choice and civil rights by focusing upon the work of COYOTE (Call Off Your Old Tired Ethics), a prostitutes' rights organization in North America. It will be interesting to follow the development of prostitutes' rights organizations as a new social movement in the coming years, particularly as they develop their work, especially advocacy work linked to women's experiences, health and welfare agencies, criminal justice agencies and policy change. The European and international prostitutes' rights movement has to date had most impact in Germany, the Netherlands and North America, generating inter-agency support, backing and campaigning and lobbying for social change.

Working in multi-agency ways with women working as prostitutes is important not only in terms of having their concerns, needs and voices heard by agencies working with and for them, but also in terms of working together in democratic ways to develop women-centred change (O'Neill 1994, 1995). Moreover, it is important to work with and for young people involved in prostitution in order to develop and implement intervention strategies which help prevent the involvement of young, vulnerable and emotionally needy young people in prostitution, as well as developing strategies of harm minimization for those who will not or cannot stop working as prostitutes (O'Neill *et al.* 1995a).

At the European Whores Congress, held in Frankfurt am Main in October 1991, delegates were made aware of the legal and social situations for prostitutes in the sixteen countries attending the congress. Many whores were vociferously against young people entering prostitution who were vulnerable, emotionally needy and not really aware of their own needs around their sexuality (Drobler 1991). The women at the congress were strong and articulate, demanding the decriminalization of prostitution and the same rights, civil liberties and rights to human dignity as other workers. Indeed the Women's Committee of the European Parliament calls on member states to decriminalize prostitution, and protect the health and safety of sex workers, pointing out that the 'semi-illegal, shady background against which prostitutes operate actually encourages such abuses as prostitution under duress, degrading working and living conditions, maltreatment and murder'. The women and men attending the first European Whores Congress in Frankfurt voted on a resolution to be included in the European Social Charter, calling for the decriminalization of prostitution and for prostitution to be accepted as a profession. But, going back to the need for law reform in this country, I would not like to see us legalize prostitution and then go down the same road as many European countries as far as the human rights and civil liberties of prostitute women are concerned (see Drobler 1991).

CONCLUSION

Working *with* women is important – their voices should be heard and listened to. Standing back from personal experience and looking at the contexts and structures in which and through which people live necessitates an examination of the employment, education and training structures and possibilities for women; the system of local authority residential care and the whole concept of 'care'; the freeing-up of traditional structures and institutions which allows for greater diversity, choice and plurality in contemporary society; the oppression and domination of women by men, illustrated so tragically by the endemic nature of violence against all women but more specifically against prostitute women. In working with the complexity of women's lives feminist research is of central importance to help create the intellectual and practical spaces for women's voices to be heard and listened to. We need to engage with the depth and complexity of women's lives in order to better understand them and to address policy change.

Key considerations for future work with prostitute women now are as follows. We need further research directed at:

- developing policy changes around women's employment and the feminization of poverty;
- violence and abuse of women and children; given the fact that violence against prostitute women is endemic, they are perceived as a throwaway population;
- the relationship between routes into prostitution, homelessness, poverty and leaving local authority residential care;
- the current and future work of the prostitutes' rights movement at national, European and international levels, particularly regarding international trafficking in women and children;
- the benefits of multi-agency working groups which are woman centred and have prostitutes represented as key players in order to develop better organized networks of support to working women around health, welfare, legal, vocational/employment needs, as well as safety needs such as safe houses, information, knowledge and counselling;
- preventative work with young people at risk;
- and last but by no means least – law reform.

Engaging with the realities of women's lives within the context of social order, insecurity and social change at an everyday as well as a more global level may enable us to understand the lived relations of women working as prostitutes now and envision and work towards better futures for all women. Women working as prostitutes are ordinary women. The reflexive interrelationship between feminist thought/research, women's lived relations and policy oriented practice is a good enough place to start.

Chapter 2

Prostitute men now

Peter Davies and Rayah Feldman

INTRODUCTION

A number of writers have commented on the remarkable way in which the appearance of AIDS[1] in the early 1980s dramatized existing social conflicts and exacerbated long-standing lines of social exclusion (Altman 1986; Watney 1987; Weeks 1989). The appearance of the new syndrome and its subsequent spread within marginalized groups appeared to validate the emergent moral agenda of the 1980s (see Grover 1989; Treichler 1989). The relationship of the hegemonic culture with gay men, with drug 'ab'users, with people from Africa, with prostitutes and with all those labelled sexually promiscuous became energized and infused with new symbolic force as the metaphors of disease, corruption, decay and death were deployed to exclude and blame those most affected by HIV.

On the other hand, the appearance of the syndrome produced a positive reaction, remarkable both for its scope and its success. Early in the epidemic, the gay communities of the United States, followed by those in northern Europe and other countries, initiated and funded safer sex campaigns, sexual health interventions and promoted new models of care and support for those affected by the virus. In the mid-1980s, state responses began to emerge (see Pollack 1990 for the European pattern of response). These have generally been ambivalently received by AIDS activists. While initiating statutory sector responses to the epidemic on a scale which non-statutory bodies could not hope to match, the state is often accused of privileging research, particularly bio-medical research, over community intervention. Male sex work rarely, if ever, emerged as an issue of importance in HIV prevention campaigns, and those programmes which were put in place depended on the initiatives of individual physicians. In the UK, the most notable exception to this trend was the charity Streetwise, whose general remit for the care of street-workers in the capital was swiftly expanded to include matters of HIV transmission.

One of the main reasons for this was the multiple marginality of male sex work. In 1990, commenting on the paucity of published work before 1980, we noted that male sex work was

> marginal to two phenomena that are themselves peripheral to academic interest: prostitution and homosexuality. But, more than that, it is the potential of male homosexual prostitution to contradict current orthodoxies that guarantees its academic invisibility. . . . Because it involves a contract between two men, [it] confounds those who regard (female) prostitution as a simple rehearsal of gender inequality. Because, in some cases, the punter pays for the orgasm of the prostitute, it challenges those who would reduce prostitution to a form of consumer capitalism: mere payment for pleasure; and because it exists at all in the era of gay liberation, it embarrasses those who extol the revolutionary egalitarianism of the gay community.
>
> (Davies and Simpson 1990: 104)

We see no reason, six years on, to withdraw from this point of view. The dominant academic picture which emerged before 1980 has had an immense effect on the shaping of policy in the 1980s and in the next section we outline some of its main features.

Before HIV

From the work that was published before the 1980s, a picture has emerged of male prostitution which, we believe, lacks methodological validity and empirical basis and which, moreover, is written from a viewpoint which claims scientific dispassion but betrays a moralistic and patronising attitude towards its 'objects of study'. The problem is well illustrated by the following extract from a paper in the *American Journal of Orthopsychiatry* (the branch of psychiatry concerned with the prevention and correction of incipient mental illness) in 1974. The author writes:

> [The male homosexual prostitute] is a drifter, has a poor work history, possesses no vocational skill, is of low to average

> intelligence, comes from a deprived socioeconomic background and is below the average of educational attainment. He is a drop-out and comes from a broken home or a home in which his parents were poor models. His was a shattered family in which there was a dearth of warmth and an excess of violence and rejection. He was the victim of indifferent mothering. Most hustlers have been found to be irresponsible, immature, unstable and neurotic with a strong dislike for authority.
>
> (Coombs 1974: 784)

This summary justifies each descriptive phrase by reference to a previous piece of research. What emerges is a methodologically suspect and empirically misleading portrait. The account treats a large number of more or less idiographic, impressionistic and *ad hoc* studies as cumulative facets of an emerging picture. It is as if a composer had produced a musical composition consisting of a bar from each piece of music published in the twentieth century and claimed that it thus represented a resumé of twentieth-century composition. Such a claim could not be upheld, nor, we suggest, should Coombs's identikit portrait be accepted without critical scrutiny and empirical test.

This method of conflating comments from ethnographic work has resulted in the creation of:

> two compelling stereotypes: that of the straight hustler and that of the teenage runaway prostitute. These two portraits, often merged in a single, sorry account, dominate contemporary sociological descriptions and fuel popular and journalistic stereotypes.
>
> (Davies and Simpson 1990: 109)

These pictures derive primarily from the work of Reiss (1961), Butts (1947) and in this country Harris (1973) and Lloyd (1979). Of these, Reiss has certainly been the most influential. He describes a group of heterosexually identified young men engaging in prostitution and characterizes the norms of the peer group which allows them to reconcile a heterosexual self-image with homosexual activity. These include an emphasis on the financial rewards of the work and a denial of physical pleasure from the sex; a disdain and even hatred for the punter and a restriction of sexual activity to the insertive, masculine role in oral intercourse (Reiss 1961: 438).

This picture of the male sex worker, the rent-boy, as a young heterosexual male, suborned against his will into the lowest and vilest of practices, existing in a relationship of economic dependency and emotional antagonism with his despised but necessary clients, remains a dominant strand in many discussions of the 'problem' of male prostitution and has, as we shall discuss below, influenced both research and policy surrounding HIV.

It is worth looking in some detail at some of the features of this approach to sex work. First, we note a reluctance to believe that the rent-boy can be homosexual by preference. Indeed, such a figure is strikingly absent from the literature. In policy terms, this presupposition manifests itself in two ways: in the implicit goal of removing the young men involved from sex work and in the failure of any interventions being targeted on, or indeed developed by, the gay community to deal with the issues of sex work.

Second, it seems taken for granted that no young man would rationally choose sex work as a means of living. We have written at length elsewhere (Davies and Project SIGMA 1992; Davies *et al.* 1993) on the misuse of the concept of rationality in AIDS discourse. In this context, it is sufficient to note that sex work can, in many circumstances, be a relatively lucrative and attractive alternative when weighed against repetitive and demoralizing factory work or the ill-paid harum-scarum of the fast-food empires. In contrast, sex work can provide relatively large sums of money in a relatively short period of time. We spoke to one individual who had given up a career as a medic in order to concentrate on sex work which was, he said, more lucrative and involved far fewer hours at work. While no doubt exceptional, this anecdotal evidence serves merely to underline our basic point. From this traditional perspective of sex work as a last resort of those without alternatives, the aim of outreach or other programmes is to dissuade the sex worker from working and to return to (heterosexual) normality. From our perspective, sex work remains an alternative to other forms of work and this must be taken into consideration in outreach and other work.

Third, child sexual abuse features prominently in discussions of male sex work (see Robinson and Davies 1991: 96ff.), especially in recent years as a series of cases and associated moral panics have brought the issue to public attention. This feature also appears in discussions in two ways. On the one hand, there are those who take the youth of the men involved in sex work as a priori evidence of the assertion that prostitution is little more than formally structured abuse (Lloyd 1979). This assertion is buttressed by descriptions of young men forced into sex work and kept in thrall by violence or other threats. It would be foolish and unhelpful to deny the existence of paedophile rings or the horrific cases of such unfortunate individuals as Jason Swift, but at the same time it is unscientific and inhumane not to recognize these as unusual, indeed exceptional events which are far from the quotidian experience of most sex workers.

On the other hand, sexual abuse also appears as a key feature of the suggested aetiology of the 'prostitute personality'. The late Richie McMullen has argued strongly for an understanding of a causal link between sexual and or physical abuse as a child and prostitution. In brief, the argument posits a 'logical process' from receiving gifts and/or money as 'reward' for suffering abuse as a child, through a process of self-legitimation in which he persuades himself of his complicity in and enjoyment of the abuse, to a position in which he 'allows himself to abuse others and/or set himself up for further abuse' (McMullen 1988: 40). West's recent work (1992) has shown no empirical basis for this contention and we have elsewhere doubted the logic of the argument, commenting on the easy and convenient aetiological linkage between two social 'problems' (Robinson and Davies 1991: 97). By discussing and 'explaining' the one in terms of the other – prostitution is a consequence of abuse – and confining the awful prospect of same-sex child abuse within an identifiable group of 'deviants', two social evils are conveniently simplified and collapsed. It would be wrong to deny the reality of child sexual abuse and its terrible consequences for the survivors. On the other hand, we believe that the attempt to reduce the one to the other is detrimental to an understanding of both.

At the heart of this traditional discourse of male prostitution is the figure of the powerless prostitute. He is, in this account, trapped by personality defects, childhood traumata or economic destitution in a cycle of penury, prostitution and self-loathing. It then follows that the aim of outreach or other programmes directed at these young men is to allow them to give up prostitution and return to some other way of life. This may be achieved in a number of ways, but all are inherently prescriptive. They focus on the inability of the individual to make the right choice: that is, not to engage in sex work.

An alternative view of sex work has emerged from within feminism. For some years women in sex work and others have sought to redefine the nature of prostitution. This work has emerged from a feminist analysis of the role of sex in general. At the heart of this tradition is an attempt to replace discussion of 'prostitution', with its connotations of deviance and sleaze, with the idea of sex work. In so doing, it attempts to render sex work as part of a continuum of sexual relations with men (see, for example, Barry 1979). It argues that the difference between prostitution and marriage – in its traditional form – is one of degree not of essence. In both cases, women are rendered relatively powerless in relation to men and enmeshed in a nexus of financial and moral dependency. It also emphasizes the economic aspect of prostitution, what people do, rather than the pathological or proto-psychiatric, what they are.

Perhaps because of its feminist origin, perhaps because of the peculiar nature of male sex work, there is no evidence of this perspective having any impact on male sex work until recently.[2] Shorn of its feminist specificities, this perspective makes the logical distinction between sex work and destitution. It recognizes and highlights the fact that the literature and most discussion of male sex work concentrates on the conjunction of these two features: looks only at the homeless, drifting or otherwise 'chaotic' young man on the streets of the large cities. It then counterpoises this with the existence of a flourishing market in sex carried out by individuals who do not in any way correspond to this stereotype (see Davies and Simpson 1990: 113ff.; Robinson and Davies, 1991: 99ff.; Hickson *et al.* 1994; also Marotta *et al.* 1988, for American examples). Noting that there are many who carry out sex work in congenial circumstances and with control over their lives and work, it argues that this is a possible aim for all those who find themselves involved in sex work. Better, they argue, to work from a flat with the ability to choose customers than from the street-corners with desperation. Having said that however, it is naive to suggest that every young man selling sex on the streets or at railway stations is capable of or wants to continue in sex work, however salubrious.

With this basic perspective, a different set of policy preferences from that associated with the traditional view emerges. These seek the decriminalization of sex work and, more broadly, its rescue from stigmatization. More specifically, it identifies the need to make sex workers better at their jobs (see Kooistra and Hazenkamp 1992). This involves a number of specific agenda. First, it rejects removal from sex work as the only or the best solution in all cases. Second, it recognizes the importance of punter-free spaces as a means to develop ways to organize their own work in as congenial manner as possible. Third, it recognizes that the aim of programmes for and by sex workers is to enable them to 'do as little as possible for as much money as possible', that is to exploit the market position that they have. This involves the encouragement of existing skills and the empowerment of individuals.

We find ourselves more convinced by the latter standpoint, in that it identifies a set of solutions which increase the choices available to those involved in sex work while recognizing the difficulties they face. In so doing, it diverts attention from the pathologizing and demeaning search for the 'prostitute personality' and towards the experience of sex work as the result of choices made by the individuals concerned, often in circumstances of stress and difficulty.

The impact of AIDS

The emergence of AIDS and the identification of the modes of transmission of HIV have led to a great deal of research on rates of HIV infection among female and, to a lesser extent, male sex workers in various cities around the world (e.g. Chiasson *et al.* 1988; Coutinho *et al.* 1988; Elifson *et al.* 1988, Tirelli *et al.* 1988). We prefer to prescind from detailed comment on these findings, since it seems a dubious and unscientific undertaking to compare the rates of HIV positivity in populations that are culturally diverse, from samples that vary in representativeness and in countries at different stages of the epidemic, as if the label 'prostitute' were a universal category with specific physical potentials for infection rather than a socially and culturally bound and constrained set of social and sexual practices and relationships. We are, therefore, dubious of attempts such as that of Darrow (1991) to quantify the state of the epidemic world-wide by comparison of these rates.

While a great deal of research proceeds with the explicit or implicit aim of quantifying the risk posed by sex workers to the general population, other work has concentrated on the minimization of risk to sex workers (see for example, Kinnell 1991). Similarly, many, if not most, health promotion projects promote the idea that unsafe sex consists of a particular behaviour or set of behaviours which have to be eradicated from the sexual repertoire. Where men having sex with men are concerned, anal intercourse is the behaviour most frequently and, given its high risk of transmission, rightly targeted activity. However, as we have elsewhere sought to argue (Davies and Weatherburn 1991, Davies *et al.* 1992), at the individual level, such monolithic assessments of risk are neither actual nor realistic nor always helpful features of sexual behaviour. While some individuals always and in every circumstance choose to avoid high-risk behaviour, there are many others who choose not to do so. The most common response to this behaviour among behavioural scientists is to emphasize its irrationality and to recommend programmes which will ensure that the individuals involved make the 'right' decision, that is to avoid the behaviours entirely. We prefer a more radical approach, believing that individuals make complex assessments of the risk involved in a particular encounter or within a particular relationship, not on the basis of a sterile weighting of the benefits of sex in that context against the likelihood of infection and the disadvantages attendant upon it, but rather on the basis of a number of heuristic, contingent weightings, some of which may be more appropriate than others. In general, we believe that many gay and bisexual men have evolved risk-minimization strategies which involve rational, well-informed and sophisticated decisions about their behaviour (for a detailed discussion of these points see Davies *et al.* 1993: Ch. 5).

At the heart of this approach is a belief in the validity of the choices made by individuals to engage in sex work and to continue to do so. We record our conviction that the aim of policy should be to extend the range of choices available. This works both on the level of the individual encounter: assuring that the choice between getting fucked in a warm bed and not getting fucked and sleeping rough is one faced by as few individuals as infrequently as possible. It also works on the wider level of lifestyle. The choice of sex work should be validated in a way that allows those who wish to do so to withdraw and those who wish to continue to work to do so with greater security and subsequent autonomy.

The role of HIV prevention is subsidiary to this main project, but greatly enhanced by this perspective. Male sex workers are a group placed at potential risk of coming into contact with HIV in the pursuit of their work. The actual risk attached to a particular individual will, of course vary with the pattern of his sexual behaviour. In general the greater the number of times he has anal intercourse, the greater the risk. The use of condoms for anal intercourse, while reducing the risk to both partners, does not, despite popular beliefs to the contrary, eradicate the risk. Smaller risks attach to the ingestion of semen, while a pattern of work that consisted solely of masturbation would seem to carry little or no risk of infection, however many clients are involved.

The degree of exposure of an individual will depend on the actual mix of practices in his repertoire. Among female sex workers in London, there is a concentration on masturbation as the primary means of 'relief'. To this extent, sex work carries with it a relatively low risk of exposure. Day (1989) has gone on to suggest that the main risk of HIV infection to female workers is through sex with non-paying partners (who may also be pimps) and through injecting drug use.

This discussion has shown that the empirical literature has a limited amount of information to divulge on the ways in which young men who sell sex live their lives – and much of that is coloured by an unhelpful, tacit moral agenda. Even less is known about the ways in which these young men currently cope with the need to avoid HIV transmission and in what ways future health promotion initiatives might enhance their abilities to do so. It was in this situation that we were asked by the Department of Health in 1992 to report on the working practices of young men who sell sex, paying particular attention to the implications of those practices for HIV prevention campaigns.

THE STUDY

In 1992, as part of this study, we interviewed a number of male sex workers in South Wales. We were concerned that previous work on this group of men had been concentrated in metropolitan areas, particularly London (indeed on one part of London) and this might have led to an unusual (possibly unique) state of affairs being taken as representative of matters across the country. Our informal contacts had convinced us that significant though small marketplaces existed in many other smaller cities and towns. South Wales was chosen as a site since we had previously undertaken research there and had already made some contacts with workers. We used a combination of methods, ranging from non-participant observation, through semi-structured interviews to, in the later stages of the project, a formal questionnaire, from which the results in the following section are drawn.

Demographics

We describe first the characteristics of the group of young men we spoke to, then move on to consider salient features of their careers as sex workers and their current experiences and practices.

The average age of the men was slightly under 18, with a range from 15 to 23 . There was a slight under-representation of older men, but not markedly so. Although the reported ages may be different from real ages (on a couple of the interview schedules the interviewer has indicated his belief that the boy is younger than he has claimed), there did not seem to be large numbers of very young men or boys involved in this scene. It is significant, however, that some 97 per cent were below the (then) legal age of consent for male homosexual sex.

The young men lived in a number of towns and cities in South Wales. Twenty-six came from Cardiff and a further seven from the Barry-Penarth cluster to the south of the city. Ten came from the Rhondda and other valleys to the north. Fourteen lived in Newport/Cwmbran and nine in Swansea, the other two major conurbations in the region. Seven came from Bridgend and four from Neath, relatively large towns between the cities of Cardiff and Swansea. Two came from Abergavenny, a market town some considerable distance from the industrial belt. Only one was presumptively homeless, claiming to live 'around and about'.

Thirty-eight of the young men (some 47 per cent) lived with their parents and another seventeen (21 per cent) with a male partner in a flat or house. Sixteen (20 per cent) lived alone in a flat or bedsit and six (7 per cent) in shared accommodation. Three were living in squats. (One missing datum.) While we do not have details on the arrangements for living together, this picture does not at first sight appear to be one of homelessness.

Some of these young men work in their home towns while others prefer to travel to the more anonymous larger cities. This tends to confirm evidence from our field-work that sex workers move from city to city, along the main train routes. Thus there is a natural movement within South Wales to Cardiff, the largest city, and from the area as a whole to Bristol, Birmingham and London.

There is also some movement to Amsterdam and, while this is organized, we have had no evidence of coercion.

Fifteen of the workers are still at school and a further fifteen have no formal educational qualifications. Forty-one claim to have CSE qualifications, a further eight GCSEs; two of these are studying for A levels, and there are five with A levels, two of whom are students in higher education. Eighteen (22 per cent) were looking for a job at the time of interview and thirty (37 per cent) were currently signing on. Fifty-seven (70 per cent) came from working-class backgrounds according to their own definitions of the class status of their father's job. The fathers of a further three (4 per cent) were unemployed. Fourteen (17 per cent) were middle class by their own definition. While this seems a relatively fair reflection of the class composition of industrial South Wales, it does not accord with the idea of these people being drawn from the 'underclass'.

Patterns of disclosure are important in that they give some clue to the ways in which HIV-relevant information and other initiatives can be channelled effectively. None of the workers had told their parents that they were doing sex work, although thirty-two (40 per cent) had told them that they had sex with men. Only four had told brothers or sisters that they worked. More surprisingly, a minority of the participants (7; 9 per cent) thought that other sex working friends did not know that they worked. This is difficult to believe, but it does point to some degree of secrecy between workers and as such a potential barrier to programmes which foster empowerment and/or peer norm enforcement programmes. The number who had non-working friends who knew they worked was only twenty (25 per cent), while forty-seven (58 per cent) were out to these friends about their sexual preference.

Career

The interview did not deal in detail with personal histories or moral careers. Participants were asked, however, to recall their first experience with a punter, that is to recall their entry into sex work. Replies were recorded from sixty-three young men.

McMullen (1988) has argued that sexual abuse in childhood or adolescence is an important, or, on one reading, the most important factor in the creation of a male sex worker. Only five (6 per cent) of the respondents reported abuse at ages ranging from 7 to 14. Another nine refused to answer this question and, in some cases, the terms in which this was done suggests a traumatic memory. The accounts are similar and moving.

> The first time ever I was 7 years old. It was my step father who sexually abused me and he used to give me sweets and toys to shut me up. So I suppose he was the first punter. It's through that bastard I'm on the streets selling myself now.

> The first time I got paid was by my step father; I was 12 years old. He used to give me money not to tell my mother that he was playing around with me. I suppose I should have said something, told somebody, but I was scared.

These data, however harrowing, must be treated with caution. On the one hand, the interview was not a situation in which a matter as traumatic as childhood abuse could easily be raised. We must therefore suspect under-reporting. Indeed, many of those who have recounted other experiences in answer to this question may also have been subject to abuse. But in the absence of information on the incidence of abuse in the population at large, any conclusions about causation or predisposition must be tentative at best.

The predominant figure in the recollections of the first experience is the recognition of an economic opportunity, though the dimensions of this are many. For a small number, a conscious decision is taken to work. For example:

> My present boyfriend introduced me to one of his punters. . . . We'd . . . decided to live together. But we had no money. So we decided that I would do punters like him and we'd pool the money until we got enough to pay a deposit on a flat.

> We had recently moved into a flat together and were finding we could afford rent, gas, electricity, food but we had little left for going out or saving for a holiday. So we discussed how we could earn extra money and as a joke at first said let's go on the game. We discussed this further and said we'd give it a try but wanking only. The first night we tried we did three punters each – that was £30 in total. Now we try to do five or six and we are saving for a holiday in Tunisia.

Others found out about the possibilities of earning money from others who earned money in that way:

One of my friends in school told me when we were wanking together that he got paid for wanking some men, so I said I'd go along with him.

My brother is gay and he always seemed to have money. One night I followed him and watched what he was doing. I told him what I'd done a few days later.

When I was 16 I went to a pub with a pal and he kept going to the toilet and coming back with money. He told me he was wanking old queens for £5 a go. He said it was easy money so I had a go.

Many, however, recall their 'first time' as part of the experimentation of youth. Central to this set of responses is the realization that what gave pleasure could also earn cash or goods.

I was 14 years old and was out fishing with an older boy. . . . He said he'd give me ten Embassy if I wanked him off. I agreed. I suppose indirectly he was my first punter as prior to that I'd done it for nothing.

I was in a public toilet and a boy came over and asked me if I wanted business. . . . I let him wank me and gave him £2. I thought it was an easy way to make money so I tried it myself and it worked. I've been doing it a couple of times a week since then.

Also noticeable is the fact that the first punter is often of the same age, or slightly older, than the boy himself. They speak of 'a boy', 'an older boy', 'older boys in school' and so on. Others have been approached by older men, usually referred to as 'old queens':

I was about 13 years old. I've always known I was gay and I used to go shopping for an old queen who lived beside us. . . . One day . . . he asked if I would like to earn some extra money and . . . I agreed to go there on a Saturday to do the garden. When I got there he was reading dirty books. He showed me some pictures and said he used to have a 'young friend' who called to see him to wank him for £5.

I used to visit an older guy (about 55) and he used to give me money to touch me up. I think he's dead now.

I was 16 years old. An old queen came up to me and I thought 'If he wants it badly enough he can pay for it.' I told him it would cost him £5 for a wank. Silly old bugger gave me £5 and I wanked him off.

While these were clearly significant events for the young men involved, it is important not to attribute causal force to them without further discussion. Doubtless many other boys and young men have been given or offered money for sex at one time or another. These young men have developed that insight, made use of that knowledge in a particular way. Their choice to become sex workers, to exploit that opportunity, is a logically separate decision. One worker recalled the importance of his first punter in making him a good sex worker:

> First punter was an old queen. . . . It was obvious that she was past her best so I agreed to go to her house the following day. I arrived to find that she'd prepared a lovely meal. After the meal she wanted me to stay. I said no, the agreement was that I would fuck her. She said she would give me £10, I said I wanted £15. She gave me £15 and I went with her into the bedroom. I fucked her and then felt guilty for taking the money so I gave her £10 back and said I'd keep the £5 to pay for my taxi. She told me I was a nice boy but silly. She then told me how she'd once been beautiful and had made money but that she'd been sensible and saved it, and that I shouldn't let sentiment come into business. I learned a lot from that old queen, who is now a friend, non-sexual, and I have learned to pick and choose punters who will pay. What she taught me has stood me in good stead.

There is no indication in the data that these young men found then or find now their older clients despicable, as Reiss (1961) claims his interviewees viewed their clients. The dominant figure is, as we have noted, one of financial advantage or compensation for a sexual contact that would otherwise not occur.

> There's always a few old queens in the club who are grateful to pay for a quickie, so I make a point of pulling three or four on a Saturday night, which pays for my night out.

In general, the relationship between worker and client appears symbiotic, ranging from the affectionate to the instrumental. In a few cases, however, violence or bloody mindedness on the part of the client is noted by workers:

> It [the sex] was over in a couple of minutes. He gave me a £20

> note and when I got out of the car to get back in the front the bastard drove off and left me.
>
> I took his zip down and started to laugh. His prick was so little I could hardly get hold of it. He thumped me in the face and kicked me in the balls. Then the bastard took his fiver back and left me on the ground.

These are, it must be stressed, isolated and atypical events in the accounts that we have collected.

Work

The traditional account has the worker forced to engage in an activity that he dislikes for the sake of money. This hypothesis is not supported by these data. Only two of the workers said that sex work was something which they disliked doing but needed the money. Most (35; 43 per cent) thought of it as a part-time job, and another five (6 per cent) as a 'hobble' (Welsh vernacular for moonlighting). On the other hand, only eight (10 per cent) said that the work was something that they liked doing. Most were indifferent, twenty-four (30 per cent) saying that it was something that they didn't mind doing and got paid for. Three of them saw it as a full-time job and another three as a hobby.

Affirmed identities were fairly evenly split between 'rent-boy' (27; 33 per cent), male prostitute (23; 28 per cent), with sex worker being favoured by fourteen (17 per cent). Other terms were put forward by another sixteen (20 per cent). These included the idea of 'supplying a service', 'fulfilling a need', 'giving the public a service' (4; 5 per cent) and the idea that this was 'just a job' (2; 3 per cent). Three saw it as 'having fun'.

Working patterns seem to vary greatly. Sixteen (20 per cent) work every day and similar numbers a four (16; 20 per cent) or five (17; 21 per cent) day week. Another group (11; 13 per cent) works only two days a week. One worker makes a fixed sum of money per week and then stops.

Sex

Seventy-eight (96 per cent) of the young men interviewed had had sex with a punter in the month before interview. Of those who had done so, the average number of punters in the month before interview was thirty-one, about one per day on average.

Thirty-one (38 per cent) had not had anal intercourse with punters in the month before interview. In some cases, this is a conscious decision, made for reasons of HIV:

> I don't fuck with punters, I'm shit scared of getting AIDS or VD.
>
> I don't fuck with punters, I'm too scared of getting AIDS.
>
> I don't fuck or suck punters. I'm too aware of HIV and Hep.B.

for reasons of personal dislike:

> Have only tried to fuck once. It hurt too much so never again.
>
> Only once let someone fuck me. Never again. It hurt too much.

or because of an agreement within a relationship:

> I work alongside my boyfriend and we have an agreement not to fuck punters.
>
> Don't fuck with punters, only girlfriend.

This set of reasons is remarkably similar to that given by men in the SIGMA research (Hickson *et al.* 1994) for engaging or not engaging in anal intercourse.

For those who did engage in anal intercourse, the average (mean) number of punters with whom fucking occurred was eighteen in the month before interview, which must, by any criteria, be regarded as high. By comparison, the average man in the SIGMA survey will have had one such partner in the same time period.

Separately, participants were asked to recount in detail where and when they had sex in the previous week. Apart from the detailed information this gives, the exercise also allows some reliability checking on the estimates of partner numbers. The total number of sessions was 523 for 80 people The average number is thus almost exactly seven, which is remarkably consistent with the estimates of partner numbers.

Thirty-seven of the young men had regular clients whom they had met in the month before interview, and seventy-seven had met casual punters. Distinctive patterns of behaviour emerge between these types as shown in Table 2.1.

While the majority of sessions with casual punters involved only masturbation and 10 per cent anal intercourse, the pattern with

Table 2.1

	Regular		*Casual*	
Service	*Number (%)*	*Price £*	*Number (%)*	*Price £*
Masturbation	0	–	253 (62)	5
Oral	6 (6)	4	113 (28)	5
Anal	80 (85)	17	41 (10)	17
Corp. punish.	8 (9)	23	0	

regular punters is quite different, with 85 per cent of sessions involving anal intercourse. Masturbation (solely) did not occur with regular punters. Corporal punishment, though very rare, also was confined to regular partners.

The patterning of practices with different types of partner points to an important conclusion. While it seems to be the case that there is, on the one hand, a group who do not engage in anal intercourse for a set of coherent reasons, it is not the case that the group which do engage do so because they are stupid, feckless or that they deny their susceptibility to HIV infection. Because the anal intercourse is patterned by relationship, it indicates that decisions are being made at the level of the encounter or of the relationship. While it may be the case that these decisions are unwise, even in some cases foolhardy, the fact that they are decisions needs to be taken into account when health promotion programmes are considered. Rather than seek to isolate and correct the deficiencies that lead individuals to engage in 'unsafe' behaviour, the process of decision-making needs to be identified, recognized and encouraged.

Although the average figure is shown in Table 2.1, the commonest cost of a fuck was £20 (63/121) or £15 (37/121). A wank was a fairly standard £5, which was the same modal price as oral sex. It is noticeable, however, that despite the difference in repertoire, the prices charged for services to regular and to casual punters do not seem to differ. It may be (and there is evidence in the participant observation data to support this) that other forms of reward are forthcoming from regular punters, such as drinks or other payments not directly related to specific sexual services: a sort of retainer fee. The prices charged and the pattern of work noted in the section above indicate clearly that sex work is not, for these young men, a full-time and financially secure job. As they themselves recognize, it is, at best, a part-time or interstitial occupation.

Non-paying sexual partners

Fifty-nine (73 per cent) of those interviewed reported a non-paying male partner during the month before interview. Of those with partners, the average number of partners was two. The relatively high proportion of men with male sexual partners does not accord with the conventional account's contention that sex workers are heterosexual. Indeed, only eight (10 per cent) of the workers had sex with a female partner in the month before interview. Forty of the fifty-nine men with non-paying male partners in the month reported that they had anal sex with all of them. Twenty-three (28 per cent) had a boyfriend, while only six (7 per cent) had a girlfriend. Two-thirds of regular partners (of either gender) knew that the worker 'did punters'.

Condoms

It is illuminating to consider differences in the pattern of condom use between regular and casual punters and regular and casual non-paying partners.[3]

Table 2.2 Number of sex workers (N) reporting, and frequency (f) of, anal intercourse with and without condoms

	Casual client		*Regular client*		*Regular partner*		*Casual partner*	
	N	*f*	*N*	*f*	*N*	*f*	*N*	*f*
Insertive	4	16	9	32	15	26	10	23
Ins. and condom	4	17	1	3	1	10	1	2
Receptive	37	450	27	255	16	40	12	36
Rec. and condom	21	153	9	38	0	0	2	3

From Table 2.2, a number of observations can be made. First, the proportion of sessions involving receptive intercourse is 84 per cent for paying partners but only 53 per cent for non-paying partners. This indicates a preponderance of that mode in paying encounters. More germanely, condoms have been used in 31 per cent of sessions involving punters but in only 7 per cent of sessions with non-paying partners. This tends to confirm findings in other studies, which indicate the symbolic importance of unprotected penetrative sex in the context of affective relationships.

Taking the frequency data, the probability of a condom being used with a regular non-paying partner is .13, while with a casual non-paying partner it is .08 (odds ratio = 1.7). This is counter-intuitive and may be due to the small numbers involved, only three young men in total.

The probability of a condom being used with a regular client is .125, while with a casual client it .27 (odds ratio = 2.6). While this result is in the right direction, the overall proportion of condom use in both cases remains lower than might be expected or is desirable.

Thirty-one (38 per cent) of the participants claimed to be carrying condoms when interviewed but only seventeen (21 per cent) always carried them while working, while another fifty-three (64 per cent) sometimes did so. Such figures need to be treated sensibly. The assumption that the workers should always be doing so depends on an assumption that fucking is to be a part of the repertoire. This need not be so. If a worker does not do anal intercourse, the need for condoms is less salient. More interesting is the finding that, on the last occasion that anal intercourse occurred with a punter, the worker provided the condom in fifty-seven (70 per cent) cases, while the punter did so in only eight (10 per cent) (remainder, not applicable). The most commonly cited source of supply for condoms was a machine (58 mentions), from an outreach worker (19), the STD clinic (17) and the chemist (13) being the next most popular. The family planning clinic (8) is slightly more popular than the old favourite, the barber (2).

Use of services

Only one of those we spoke to was not registered with a GP. This seems to be a feature of the population and the fact that these are not indigent youngsters but settled individuals with permanent addresses. To the extent that this pattern is true of sex work in the non-metropolitan centres, the provision of suitable services through GPs needs to be considered.

Many people would see the GUM clinic as the natural place for these people to make contact with the statutory sector, though this does not accord directly with the experience of those we interviewed. Three-quarters of the men (61; 75 per cent) had not attended an STD/GUM clinic, although the twenty who had ever done so had done so in the last year.

Having said that, only one of those twenty had told the clinic staff that he was a sex worker. Of those who had attended, all except one said that they had been treated 'OK' in the clinic, though whether this is due to an adequate service or to low expectations remains to be seen.

The number of reported STD infections is very – indeed almost incredibly – low. The only infections are crabs, reported by seven of those interviewed.

HIV and AIDS

There was a general vagueness about sources of information on HIV and AIDS, with most workers (38; 47 per cent) saying that all the listed sources were useful and eight (10 per cent) saying that none were. Of the single sources, outreach programmes were specifically mentioned by nine (11 per cent) of the workers. Only three (4) per cent mentioned other sex workers and none mentioned punters. This suggests that outreach work is currently useful, although there is not a targeted programme in the area. Even when specifically questioned about punters as a source of information on HIV and AIDS, only one of the participants said that (a) punter(s) had given him information about HIV and safer sex. Similarly, only one reported that he gave information to his punters. These pieces of information can be interpreted in two ways: either that safer sex is a taken-for-granted part of the culture and need not be talked about or that the punter–worker relationship is not the place where such conversations take place.

Seven (9 per cent) of those interviewed said that they had made changes to their sexual behaviour since HIV. It should be remembered, however, that for most if not all of these young men, AIDS has been a feature of their lives since they became sexually active. Even the oldest would have been 13 in 1981. The notion of change therefore is of less salience and the finding certainly does not indicate, of itself, a denial of the risk of HIV.

Only one averred an intention to change, a decision that must be seen in the context of current behaviour. It may be though that fatalism or a sense of 'it's been OK so far so I can carry on' underpins this attitude. Perhaps the most poignant answer to this question was that given by an 18-year-old who turned out to be seropositive. He simply said that it was 'too late'. Twenty four (30 per cent) of those we spoke to had had an HIV test result, six of whom had had more than one. Three were positive. It would, however, be scientifically absurd and morally irresponsible to base an estimate of prevalence on these small figures.

Drug use

Drug use among this group was relatively low. The most widely used drug of choice was ecstasy, taken by fourteen (17 per cent), though this was something which they did, on average, only about once a week. Unsurprisingly, marijuana was the most common drug, taken by twelve (15 per cent) of the young men, for whom this was a daily event. Indeed, they said that they smoked, on average, three spliffs a day. Next most common was cocaine, taken by just five (6 per cent), once or twice a week. Heroin and methadone were each daily habits for two young men and a further two took solvents a few times per week. Speed was taken weekly by another two and one respondent reported downers and another PCP daily.

Sixty-seven (83 per cent) of the young men interviewed reported having drunk alcohol in the week before interview and these had averaged an intake of 25 units in this period. This compares with a recommended intake of 21 units, but is probably in line with consumption levels of young men in South Wales. Thirty-eight (47 per cent) smoked 25 cigarettes per day on average.

SUMMARY CONCLUSIONS

We chose to begin our research in South Wales, but there is no a priori reason to suppose that the towns and cities of this area are significantly different from other non-metropolitan cities and towns in the United Kingdom. We must tentatively conclude, therefore, that all towns and cities in the United Kingdom will have populations of sex workers similar in number to those found in the towns and cities of this region.

Having said that, there is every reason to believe that London in particular, and the metropolitan areas in general, will have populations of sex workers that differ from those of provincial cities and towns, partly in scale, because a larger city will (ceteris paribus) generate a larger market, with the opportunities for specialization and market segmentation that this allows. We may also presume that the greater in-migration to these centres by young, indigent and homeless young men will have an effect on the market.

We have interviewed eighty-one young men in South Wales who are currently engaged in sex work. While we suspect that these comprise a large fraction of the more or less regular workers in the area, it must be recognized that an unknown number of more casual workers will also be involved. The existence of such casual participants in the market is problematic for the traditional school of thought with its emphasis on the 'prostitute personality'. The notion of sex work makes it easier to appreciate the possibility of relatively casual participation in the market, but it does not make easier the practical process of finding such workers – either for research such as this or for outreach programmes – whose attachment to the scene and relationships with other workers are temporary and unpredictable.

The total size of these populations, while individually small, is large by international standards. Research in Amsterdam, generally regarded as one of the main European centres of the sex trade, estimated that sixty boys were working in that city during the winter period (van de Lagemaat 1986), although numbers increased during the warmer months. If this is the case, then the population in an 'ordinary' area such as South Wales approximates to that in the extraordinary setting of Amsterdam.

Sex work in this area is almost completely articulated around the 'street' scene. One young man is maintained in a house by his regular punter and we have noted one other who advertises his services in the gay press. Attempts to contact him have, however, proved unproductive. The lack of a substantial non-street sector means that the possibility of pursuing sex work as a more organized business operation is less apparent to these young men. This choice may attract only a small proportion of the young men involved, but it is one that should be available to them as an option. There is some evidence from the participant observation that some young men are recruited to move to work in Amsterdam. Our reports indicate that this is presented and accepted as a business proposition and there is no evidence of coercion. Indeed, we have no reason to suspect that any form of 'pimping' or other control is present in this area.

Nearly all young men in this work in this area are below the age of male homosexual consent. While relations with the police are generally low-key, the possibility of prosecution is always present. During the research period, a case was prosecuted at the Cardiff Crown Court involving one young man who had given to the police the names of men with whom he had had sex while under 21. This law is widely disregarded by those whom it affects and, in practice, by some statutory agencies such as GUM clinics; its existence must remain, nevertheless, a potential barrier to effective action by other agencies.

The number of young men from within the gay communities of South Wales suggests that these may form an important point of first contact for many on the sex work scene, though the presumptions that all male sex workers are gay or that gay men are necessarily the best people to undertake work with this group should not be accepted without examination.

There is no evidence in these data to support the contention that drug users take to sex work to provide the money to support their habits, nor does such evidence emerge from the participant observation phase of the research. Drug use in this group appears relatively low and to take the forms that might be expected.

Excessive alcohol consumption does not seem to be a feature associated with this group as a whole nor with individual episodes of unsafe sexual behaviour.

The data include some episodes of sexual abuse in childhood or adolescence, which the survivors identify as a factor in their eventual decision to engage in sex work. While the data will not support the conclusion that the connection is causal, the theme is prominent enough to warrant attention. The importance of this presumed aetiology in the literature probably outweighs its significance in work with this group of young men. The presumption is, first, that abuse in childhood or early adulthood predisposes the young man to sex work and, second, that it creates a feeling of alienation and powerlessness which renders the individual powerless in encounters with clients. The data we have collected do not address in detail the question of aetiology or moral career. We fear that to concentrate on this aspect of life is unhelpful. We have already recorded our conviction that the linkage between the two phenomena (male sex work and abuse) appears morally convenient. We fear that the widespread acceptance of this aetiology may lead to undesirable consequences. First, we fear the substitution of a correlation by a necessary precursor. We fear that some workers may insist that admitting abuse is a necessary first step towards cure or acceptance of their status. Second, while accepting the reality of abuse and its consequences, it may be the case that exploring these events will be an important catharsis. Third, we suspect that over-emphasis on this aetiology encourages individuals to see themselves as powerless: the 'victims' of circumstance. In conclusion then, we suggest that the connection between the two phenomena is pertinent but neither necessary nor necessarily important to the present circumstances of the individual.

The predominant feature in the accounts given by these young men of their entries into sex work is the recognition of an economic opportunity. Their continued work and the income it generates finances various aspects of different lifestyles, but the general picture is that it is a source of relatively small amounts of extra cash to participate in a street lifestyle. This general picture should not, however, obscure the wider canvas of differing motives, rationales and the modes of work that these entail.

Relations with punters range from the loving to the violent. The young man kept by his lover/punter has a relationship that is difficult to distinguish from many which would not be claimed as commercial, while we have reproduced some accounts of the violence encountered by the workers. These descriptions form the extremes of a continuum, the majority of which is characterized by a more or less hasty, agreed and accepted exchange of money and sex.

In the participant observation we have noted the symbiosis that seems to characterize the relationship between the young men and some, at least, of their clients. These data give some support to the contention that there exists a sub-set of clients – some who may themselves have been workers in the past – from whom the culture of sex work can be learned. This relationship is a potentially important focus of the health promotion programme, though one particularly bedevilled by the illegality of any actual sexual contact.

The patterns of work reported also vary considerably between individuals. It would seem that for very few of these young men is sex work an organizing principle of their lifestyle. Rather, it is something that figures more or less prominently alongside other occupations, preoccupations and expectations. For a few, particularly those still living at home and attending school, it is a weekend pastime. For others it is a source of income with a precisely identified purpose.

Sexual behaviour, particularly safer sex, follows a complex pattern. A third of the group (37 per cent) do not engage in anal intercourse with punters, and these appear to be older than the others. Of those that do so, the average number of punters is high. The most noticeable patterning of activity, however, is by type of relationship. It is clear that fucking is more common with non-paying partners than with punters, and within both these groups, with regulars than casuals. The same pattern can be distinguished in condom use. Although condoms feature as the most important feature of 'safe sex' as defined by these young men, few carry or use them.

The relationship of these young men with health care providers is not ideal. While most used one or more of the services available, few felt able to disclose to those in authority that they were workers. This suggests that the statutory sector is not currently constituted in a way that encourages the specific concerns of sex workers to be addressed.

Part II

Social and legal status

Chapter 3

The legal regulation of prostitution
a human rights issue

Susan Edwards

INTRODUCTION

In this chapter I shall review current legal efforts in England and Wales to regulate prostitution and allied offences. This examination will be placed within the context of the competing theorizations of prostitution currently being debated in Europe and elsewhere, *inter alia* – on the one hand that prostitution is sex and on the other that prostitution is exploitation/inequality. I shall examine the influence these very different ideological constructions have had on shaping law and policy as it relates to prostitution, and will consider too the implications of these competing arguments for our domestic regulation. The 'prostitution as sex' and 'prostitution as exploitation/inequality' debate has become increasingly sophisticated in recent years, taking on a new language in efforts either to further the acceptability of prostitution within society or to heighten awareness of the inherent inequality. The prostitution issue is firmly on the human rights agenda, not only represented by a lobby arguing that it is an abrogation of fundamental human rights but represented too by the counter-claim that the right to prostitute is a fundamental human right.

THE LAW REGULATING DOMESTIC PROSTITUTION

Prostitution itself has never been a criminal offence. The law in England and Wales has focused instead on those activities which offend against 'public order and decency', i.e. solicitation. The law has, however, been decided in its prosecution of those who 'live off the earnings of prostitution' and those who 'exercise control over prostitute(s)'. This differential formulation of legal regulation on gender lines finds further expression in both law and its disparate application, illustrated by the grossly disproportionate prosecution of women engaged in solicitation (streetwalking) compared with the prosecution of men for the offence of kerb-crawling. In 1990 10,470 women were prosecuted for loitering and soliciting compared with 1,470 prosecutions of males for kerb-crawling. In 1991 the figures were 10,175 and 1,406 respectively. In 1992 there were 9,459 and 1,089 prosecutions, and in 1993, 7,912 as against 857 respectively (see *Criminal Statistics* 1990, 1991, 1992, 1993).

What amounts to prostitution?

A vagrancy offence

The legal regulation of prostitution dates back to the Justice of the Peace Act 1361 but it is the nineteenth-century legislation which is of contemporary relevance. From the Vagrancy Act 1824 and before, it was the female prostitute who was subject to control. Powers to penalize anyone acting in a 'riotous and indecent manner' were used by police to watch, charge and prosecute women on the streets (Edwards 1981a: 56–7). These powers were later extended by the Metropolitan Police Act 1839, which applied to Londoners, and the Town Police Clauses Act 1847 (s. 28, 'every common prostitute or nightwalker loitering and importuning passengers for the purposes of prostitution'), which extended these same powers to police forces in cities and towns outside the capital. The most appalling vista of state regulation and victimization of women in nineteenth-century England, when women were 'policed' as a class, is to be found in the Contagious Diseases Act(s) of 1864, 1866 and 1869 (see Walkowitz 1977). The philosophy guiding these Acts considered prostitute women as purveyors of the diseases of syphilis and gonorrhoea, and children and men who fell victim were morally blameless and in need of protection through the control of these women (Gorham 1978). Whilst no longer a vagrancy offence, the focus of legislative concern rests on prostitution as a street nuisance.

What activities are prostitution?

Prostitution has never been defined in statute; its meaning therefore is derived from common law. It is judges who have decided and continue to decide precisely what activities amount to prostitution and who can be regarded as a prostitute. In *de Munck* [1918] (1 KB 635), the leading case, prostitution involves the selling of sex 'in lewdness for payment' (although this may not necessarily include sexual intercourse). Reaffirming this definition, the court in *Webb* [1964] (1 QB 357) took the view that it matters not whether she plays the active or the passive role. In a case where the activity paid for amounted to the masturbation of male clients, the court held that it matters not: 'whether she whips the man or the man whips her'. (The position under American law is quite different as prostitution requires sexual intercourse (see *State* v. *Davis* (1959) (165 NE 2ND 504)).

Clippers

In a judgment delivered on 20 December 1993, in *R* v. *McFarlane* [1994] (2 All ER 283), in dismissing an appeal brought by a man convicted of living off immoral earnings, the court deliberated on the meaning of 'prostitute' and the accepted wisdom on what activities amounted to 'prostitution'. The appellant claimed that he was wrongly convicted since he was living off the earnings of a 'clipper' and not off the earnings of a 'prostitute'. Legal argument on his behalf sought to draw a distinction between a 'clipper' and a 'prostitute'. A prostitute, it was argued, offered services, accepted payment and provided those services, whilst a 'clipper' offered sexual services for reward and accepted payment in advance with no intention of providing those services. The issue on appeal was whether as a matter of law the judge at trial was correct to rule and direct the jury that a woman who offered sexual services, received payment and failed to provide the agreed service was in fact engaged in 'prostitution' within the meaning of s.30 of the 1956 Act. The Lord Chief Justice, Lord Taylor, in delivering the judgment of the Court of Appeal upholding the conviction of the lower court, ruled that indeed the appellant was guilty of 'living off immoral earnings'. Any difference between a clipper and a prostitute was, in the court's view, immaterial.

(I cannot agree with the decision of the Court of Appeal. Technically an offence of fraud, false pretences, obtaining money by deception, more accurately describes the activities of the 'clipper' than a prostitute, who provides a service not merely the promise of one. The man who lives off the income of a fraudster cannot properly be proceeded against for living off immoral earnings. However much the law might wish to regulate this behaviour and plug this lacuna in the present legislation, it is a matter for Parliament and not for the Court of Appeal.)

What is a prostitute?

A person who engages in sexual activity which is sold 'in lewdness for payment' (*de Munck*, *supra*), has been, in law, exclusively restricted to females. The sex-specific limitation is enunciated in *Webb* (*supra*). The might of the law has been directed against female street prostitutes, rather than women working elsewhere, or against the client or controller. Inequality is institutionalized by and through the law's definition of a prostitute as female, the control of women who are engaged in prostitution rather than the male client, and by a selective control of the street prostitute, arguably the poorest and most vulnerable, rather than other women who work, often covertly, in other areas of the 'sex industry'.

Rent law

Solicitation by males has been restricted to homosexual solicitation. The law has never entertained the possibility that males might sell their services to women or to men. The Sexual Offences Act 1967 s. 32, makes it an 'offence for a man persistently to solicit or importune in a public place for immoral purposes'. Here, the essence of the 'immoral purpose' has been taken to imply homosexuality (see *Selvey* v. *DPP* [1990] AC 304), not the offering of sexual services by heterosexual women to men. The sex-specific construction of the law was recently unsuccessfully challenged in the case of *DPP* v. *Bull* [1994] (4 All ER 411). This was an application by way of case stated by the Director of Public Prosecutions against a decision of Wells Street magistrates, that s. 1(1) of the Street Offences Act 1959 was limited to the activities of female prostitutes and excluded from its scope the similar activities of males. Lord Justice Mann and Justice Laws, presiding, dismissed the appeal, upholding the decision of the magistrates.

(In Australia in *Poiner* v. *Harris ex parte Pointer* (1986) (22 A.Crim.R. 370 (QdSCFC)) the court held that the term 'prostitution' may apply to the activities of both males and females and to both heterosexual and homosexual activities.)

Regulating solicitation

Solicitation by women, more commonly described as 'street-walking', is provided for by the Street Offences Act 1959 s. 1(1) where: 'It shall be an offence for a common prostitute to loiter or solicit in a street or public place for the purpose of prostitution.' Prior to 1959 prostitutes were prosecuted under the Vagrancy Act s. 3 (*supra*). Following the recommendations of the Wolfenden Committee (1957), a cautioning system already in operation in Glasgow and Edinburgh was introduced nationally, whereby police were empowered to caution women whom they considered to be soliciting on the first and second occasion, and on the third occasion of solicitation women were charged and proceeded against. This method of surveillance of first-time prostitutes was to ensure that women so cautioned had the opportunity of redeeming themselves before being branded in a court as a 'common prostitute'. Once proceeded against for an offence of 'loitering and soliciting' the cautioning system became redundant and obsolete. The result is that women with one or more previous conviction(s) find themselves under scrutiny and their mere presence on the streets often leads to further arrest and prosecution. (For a discussion of policing, see Edwards and Armstrong 1988; Edwards 1991a).

When women are charged with 'loitering and soliciting' the charge sheet is read thus, 'Miss Edwards, you being a common prostitute did loiter and solicit in Oxford Street on January 1st 1994 for the purposes of prostitution.' It is at that point that the defendant is asked: 'What do you plead?' In a criminal justice system founded on the maxim of 'innocent until proven guilty beyond reasonable doubt', it is anomalous that it is the offence of loitering and soliciting alone where an antecedent presumption of guilt is all too readily assumed. This appalling and blatant abuse of process clearly flouts even contemporary statute (see Criminal Justice Act 1991 s. 29(1); repealed Criminal Justice Act 1993 s. 66(6)). Case law prior to 1991 has held that a poor criminal record should not be regarded as an aggravating factor relevant to offence seriousness, and certainly not a factor relevant to guilt in the instant case. Given this anomalous situation it is not surprising that the percentage rate of guilty pleas for this offence is higher than for any other offence (see Edwards 1984). Several unsuccessful efforts have been made to amend the 1959 Act to revise this overtly discriminatory aspect of the legislation. Lord Chorley introduced two bills, one in 1967 and one in 1969, in an effort to amend the use of the term 'common prostitute'. In 1990 a further bill was introduced to no avail.

The vulnerability of the young

Over the decade up until 1989, when 29 per cent of prostitute women proceeded against were under 21 years of age, the involvement of young women and women under 17 years old in prostitution was increasing (Edwards 1991a). Since 1990 there has been a marginal reduction in young women proceeded against: in 1990 24 per cent, in 1991 26 per cent, in 1992 21 per cent and in 1993 20 per cent. This can be explained not by a reduction of young women turning to prostitution, but rather as a result of new police initiatives developed with social service panels whereby options other than prosecution are considered. The concern with the problem of the prostitution of young women and teenage girls, in particular juvenile prostitution, has been reflected in two recent decisions of the Court of Appeal. In the case of *Pickup* (1992) (14 Cr App R (S) 271), a middle-aged man was charged with indecent assault against a 14-year-old girl. She claimed that he had inserted his fingers and also his penis into her vagina. In his defence, he claimed that he had only inserted his finger into her vagina, which was something which he claimed he did in exchange for money. The court reduced his sentence on appeal to 9 months. In *James* (1994) (15 Cr App R (S) 100), a sentence of 18 months was upheld where a man in his 50s was convicted of indecent assault. He had fondled girls of 12, and oral sex was performed for £20. The three girls had been working as prostitutes. The Court of Appeal upheld the sentence of the Crown Court whose presiding judge in his judgment echoed the concern of the Court:

> I accept . . . that these girls were already corrupted when you became involved with them. They were already prostitutes, their own statement makes that clear. I accept also that you were not responsible for that condition . . . nevertheless, you corrupted them further. It has, on my judgment, to be made clear that child prostitution is vicious and evil, and in my judgment any man who engages in it whatever his background and circumstances, and albeit that the girls are already corrupt, already prostitutes, must go to prison. In my judgment society will be affronted by any other penalty.

Regulating the controllers – procuration and pimping

The law has also been concerned to penalize the procurer (Sexual Offences Act 1956 s. 22(1)), the pimp who lives off the earnings of prostitution (s. 30(1)) and women who exercise control over prostitute women (s. 31). Procuration, as was held by the Court in *Broadfoot* [1976] (3 All ER 753), applies to any activity which brings about the course of conduct of prostitution which the girl would not have engaged in of her own volition. Common perceptions of procuration conjure up images of pimps who frequent train stations looking to pick up vulnerable young women with a view of recruiting them into prostitution. A definition of living on the earnings of prostitution in s. 30(1), by contrast, provides: 'It is an offence for a man knowingly to live wholly or in part on the earnings of prostitution.' In interpreting this section the courts have sought to draw a distinction when sentencing the offender between the passive and coercive ponce. In *Farrugia and Others* (1979) (69 Cr App R 108) and *Hassan El-Ghazzar* (1986) (8 Cr App R (S) 182), where both defendants operated escort agencies, although there was no evidence of coercion a sentence of 2 and 1 year's imprisonment, respectively, was upheld. Section 30(1) has also been held to extend to those who supply services. However, proving the evidential element of 'knowingly' living on the earnings of prostitution has been shown to be a difficult hurdle to surmount, since the most common line of defence is that they did not know that the woman in question was a prostitute.

The Sexual Offences Act 1967 s. 5, also penalizes a man or woman for living off the earnings of the prostitution of another man, and so, for the purposes of 'living off immoral earnings', male prostitution is indirectly recognized in the law. In *Puckerin* (1990) (12 Cr App R (S) 602), the appellant had a prison sentence of 2 years reduced to 9 months. Puckerin was seen to approach young men at London railway stations and introduce them to clients. Similarly, the cases of *Connery* (1989) (11 Cr App R (S) 76) and *Hemans* (1987) (9 Cr App R (S) 25) involved convictions of men for living off immoral earnings of male prostitutes.

Women exercising control over prostitutes for the purposes of gain have been prosecuted under s. 31 of the 1956 Act. In 1975, Janie Jones received a 7-year prison sentence for 'exercising control'. The prosecution case was that the women involved were intimidated and their promise had been obtained by false pretences. It was under this section of the Act that Cynthia Payne was convicted following the discovery of her 'sorority house' ([1980] Crim LR 595). The offence of keeping a disorderly house or brothel-keeping (s. 33) has boasted such defendants as Cynthia Payne (see *Payne*, *supra*). Notwithstanding the legal efforts to penalize these 'allied' offences, prosecutions for procuration and brothel-keeping are few in comparison with annual prosecutions for streetwalking. In 1990, 482 males and 23 females were proceeded against for procuration, in 1991 346 males and 23 females, in 1992 177 males and 31 females, and in 1993 124 males and 10 females were proceeded against. Turning to brothel-keeping, in 1990 150 females and 36 males were prosecuted, in 1991 107 females and 25 males and in 1993 70 females and 20 males.

Regulating the consumers – the law of the kerb

Despite decades of agitation and mounting pressure, the punter has been the subject of prosecution only in very recent years, and even then the focus has been on the kerb-crawler, emphasizing a concern with the public nuisance of prostitution (*Street Offences Report* 1929, Wolfenden Committee 1957).

We are told that it was widely believed that the solicitation of women by men for the purpose of prostitution was indeed provided for by s. 32 of the Sexual Offences Act 1956. In *Crook* v. *Edmondson* [1966] (2 QB 81), where a man who solicited young women was prosecuted under the Sexual Offences Act 1956, s. 32, the court, in testing the application of the section, held that a male soliciting women for the purpose of prostitution did not constitute an 'immoral' purpose. Thus, it would appear to be the case that if women are soliciting this is considered for an 'immoral' purpose, but if men are soliciting women for the same end this is not an immoral purpose. The law clearly demonstrates its differential treatment of men and women in the interpretation of statute and its predilection to turn its attention away from the activity which is the object of legislation, to the person doing it, so to speak. Recent case law indicates that whether it is an immoral purpose is a matter for the jury (see *Grey* (1982) 74 Cr App R 324). In *R* v. *Dodd* (1978) (66 Cr App R 87), the words, 'Come here, I want to screw you', spoken to two 14-year-old girls, was behaviour deemed unlawful under the Sexual Offences Act 1956 s. 6(1), but only considered 'immoral' because the girls so propositioned and insulted were under the age of consent. The result has been that men have been free to solicit/importune all women of 16 years and over with impunity.

The situation is obviously most unsatisfactory. In an effort to penalize the kerb-crawler in the early 1980s, several kerb-crawlers were prosecuted under the 1361 Justices of the Peace Act. In *Hughes* v. *Holley* (1986) (86 Cr App R 130), the defendant was bound over to be of good behaviour, the court having concluded that his behaviour was offensive and contrary to standards of decency. He appealed against the magistrates' decision. Measures to penalize the kerb-crawler were met at first with a contradictory response. To the pro-kerb-crawling lobby, it seemed that at last all women, including non-prostitute women who used the streets to move to and from work, to the supermarket, to places of entertainment in the course of their everyday lives, would now have some measure of protection from unwelcome harassment by males who might accost them. Second, there were those who were concerned that criminalization of the punter would result in the further policing of marginalized men and be used as an excuse to keep watch on men in the black community; and there was a concern that prostitute women would be rendered even more vulnerable. Their vulnerability would increase since punters would be less willing to spend time in negotiations on the street, or indeed in a stationary car, about price or place, and prostitute women would have less time to 'sus' out the punter, being forced under pressure of this added surveillance to make snap judgements and accept a client they might otherwise have refused. Again support for the legislation was rallied from both the right and the left, and those who opposed the new law did so from the position that it further criminalized prostitution and put street prostitute women at risk. The Sexual Offences Act 1985 s. 1 penalized men who solicited women for the purposes of prostitution. The evidential proof required depends on the 'persistence' of the solicitation, or else solicitation in such a manner as to be 'likely to cause annoyance' to the woman or a nuisance to other persons in the neighbourhood. In the latter case such evidence was considered difficult to obtain and only to be applied in exceptional circumstances. Home Office Circular 52/1985 issued guidance on the kind of exceptional circumstances. Home Office Circular 14/1985 issued guidance on the use of a caution rather than prosecution as an alternative to the prosecution of offenders.

The Act very shortly proved to be unworkable (Edwards 1987). Police had to prove 'persistent' solicitation rather than solicitation *per se*. By direct comparison the evidential requirement for solicitation by women under the Street Offences Act does not require persistence. It was almost impossible to satisfy the test. These insuperable difficulties in application led to the introduction of a Private Members Bill on 11 May 1990 with the aim of removing 'persistently' from the Act. Alongside the evidential obstacles to effective prosecution was the unwillingness of police to prosecute men, whose only error in their view was to consort with a prostitute. Police forces preferred to use other methods of deterring prostitution and considered the exposure of men to prosecution and attendant publicity overly punitive. Police forces up and down the country developed their own local methods of dealing with the problem, ranging from informal warnings, to cautions and in some cases prosecutions. Some police officers saw themselves as moral guardians of family values offering advice to kerb-crawlers: 'What would the wife say?' 'Think about the kiddies', said one officer interviewed by the author. Kate Millet, in a footnote in *The Prostitution Papers* (1973: 87), found a similar under-enforcement of the law in the United States: 'The recent New York statute which declares the male client guilty too, in an act of female prostitution, is simply not enforced.' Of men who faced prosecution in the early days of the legislation, one of the more notorious of cases was the conviction for kerb-crawling of Colin Hart Leverton QC in 1986 (a conviction overturned on appeal). And in 1991 police in King's Cross, London, warned the former Director of Public Prosecutions, Mr Allan Green. The attendant high-profile publicity led to his resignation (Edwards 1991b). This gender politics of selective enforcement of the law extends further, even unto the difference in the evidential requirements to prove the offence of solicitation (a female-only offence) and the offence of kerb-crawling (a male-only offence), whereby prostitute women commit a crime by one act of solicitation whilst male kerb-crawlers must be cited on several occasions to satisfy the 'persistent' requirement. It is as if the state is setting its face against the weakest and most vulnerable who are selectively victimized by the law and the full force of its might. In 1989, with the Court of Appeal decision in *Paul* v. *DPP* (1990) (90 Cr App R 173), where a conviction for kerb-crawling was upheld in the High Court, the evidence tendered securing the conviction was that the defendant's behaviour was 'likely to cause a nuisance'. Although no one was in the vicinity at the time, the magistrates took into account their local knowledge of the area and, because it was residential, decided that it was reasonable to draw the assumption that the behaviour was 'likely to cause a nuisance'. The ruling in *Paul* (*supra*) meant that prosecutions were now sanctioned under the nuisance rung of the Act. This new evidential approach may have contributed to the increase in prosecutions from 220 in 1986 to 1,047 in 1989 and 1,470 in 1992, although it is curious that 1993 prosecutions have fallen dramatically to 857. It is not only the kerb-crawler but also the cruiser, that is the man who drives round red light areas watching street prostitutes and sometimes stopping his car and in a public place behaving indecently by masturbating, for example, who also creates a nuisance (see Edwards 1993a, 1993b for a discussion of punters). In *Darroch* v. *DPP* (*The Times*, 11 May 1990), it was held that the act of driving round and round a red light district does not constitute soliciting. This has left the cruiser immune from prosecution.

THE PARAMETERS OF POLITICAL DEBATE

The development of law and policy regulating prostitution is influenced by the wider philosophical and jurisprudential understanding of the problem. The debate which preceded the Street Offences Act of 1959 was moved by the question, and quite rightly, of how far the law can rightfully intervene to regulate prostitution. The debate in recent years has been reconstructed and reshaped in rather different conceptual terms. The debate works at two levels. First, there is the schism between those who argue prostitution is sex and a matter of privacy and freedom, and those who argue that prostitution is a matter of inequality and exploitation. At the second level, the prostitution-as-sex protagonists, in developing their argument further, wish to make a distinction between free prostitution, that which is freely entered into, and forced prostitution, that which is not. The advocates of prostitution as inequality and exploitation, in extending their arguments, contend that prostitution is an exploitative institution, that its existence is contrary to human dignity and, as such, is a violation of human rights. These two poles in the debate will shape the climate in which the reconstruction of legal prostitution in Europe, and possibly the UK, will take place in future years. They are arguments which we must heed.

Over the past decades the politics of prostitution has been debated by a plurality of interested factions. Right-wing moralists have been resolutely determined that prostitution must be more stringently regulated, calling for more law and punitive sanctions, more policing and more prosecution. Civil libertarians and those on the left broadly share the concern that prostitution laws are oppressive, and that they penalize women and working-class women in particular. But the solutions offered are several and competing. Some on the left argue for abolition of regulation of prostitution altogether, since the penal measures and accompanying enforcement are part of the problem. Some on the left include feminists who argue that prostitution is essentially about sexual choice, that there is a free market and that women should be free to sell themselves, prioritizing capitalism and seeing prostitution as another commodity. In this respect a distinction has been drawn between forced prostitution and free prostitution, whereby forced prostitution, which involves the exploitation of women in underdeveloped economies, is to be regulated, and free prostitution, which involves women who make a conscious decision to enter into prostitution without coercion, should be left unregulated.

Others, again on the left, are of the view that prostitution is exploitative and involves overt and covert abuse and that the way forward is to wage a war on the institutions which support prostitution. Part of this war against the institutionalization of prostitution demands a degree of criminalization of the activity, even if, regrettably, some women are penalized and some aspects of the law are unjust. Evelina Giobbe, herself a former prostitute, of WHISPER (Women Hurt in Systems of Prostitution Engaged in Revolt), and the Council for Prostitution Alternatives, two American-based groups, argue that prostitution exploits women. It is the contention of WHISPER that 'the function of the institution of prostitution is to allow males unconditional sexual access to women and children limited solely by their ability to pay for this privilege'.

Nickie Roberts (1986: 16), a former stripper writing on the 'industry' in Britain, takes a rather different view:

> Feminist anti-porn campaigners or the Mary Whitehouse brigade: it makes no difference to us. Both factions clamour for more repression and censorship at the hands of the state; both divert attention from the real issue of women's poverty in this society; and both are responsible for the increased hounding and vilification of women who work in the sex industry.

Prostitution: inequality, violence against women

For the protagonists of this conceptualization, prostitution is the institution upon which the sexual exploitation of women and children is built and it is within this framework that prostitution is discussed. Prostitution is an institution which reduces women to a sexual commodity to be bought and sold and abused. It is part of a wider systematic abuse, commodification and objectification of women as a 'sex class' and is sustained in several forms eg *inter alia* pornography. Prostitution is part of a wider violence against women perpetrated against them in peace and in plenty, in war and in poverty. This wider violence against women claims wife-beating, bride-burning, rape, incest, pornography, genital mutilation, and rape as torture, amongst its diverse forms. For MacKinnon it is precisely sexual objectification which is the central process within the dynamic of gender inequality (MacKinnon 1982: 201). For Dworkin (1989: 203) 'The sexual colonisation of women's bodies is a material reality . . . the institutions of control include law, marriages, prostitution, pornography . . . '; and for Pateman part of this colonization depends upon presenting prostitution exclusively as a private contract. She writes: 'Like other forms of capitalist enterprise, prostitution is seen as private enterprise, and the contract between client and prostitute is seen as a private arrangement between a buyer and a seller' (1989: 187).

There is nothing new in the formulation that prostitution is a form of violence against women. Engels in *The Origin of the Family Private Property and the State* (1986) characterized prostitution as a form of sexual slavery. Alexandra Kollontai in *Sexual Relations and the Class Struggle* (1978) regarded prostitution as at the heart of the woman question; speaking to women she urged them to: 'Make yourselves free from the enslavement of man.' Indeed central to the struggle for socialism is the necessity of women's freedom and equality, and freedom from male exploitation and control. Capitalism and the growth and proliferation of the capitalist 'sex industry', even in the liberal democracies of Europe, has grown to obscure the fundamental exploitation that persists as a visceral part of the institution of prostitution. There is a growing recognition that prostitution is exploitative, but such a perspective is difficult to sustain when the biggest capitalist enterprises – the media – benefit from the trade in pornography and prostitution and seek to suppress the argument of exploitation and to promote the issue of sexual freedom and choice. Prostitution is part of the new free market enterprise culture. As Kathleen Barry argues, prostitution is a part of the 'cultural climate of sadism'. This appreciation was influential in guiding the deliberations of the Meese Commission reporting on *Pornography and Prostitution* (1986: 1058) when it concluded: 'prostitution is the foundation upon which pornography is built'.

On this basis it can be observed that prostitution involves control both overt and covert. The overt forms and nature of this control are manifested by the kind of circumstances which were raised in the case of *Parker* (1985) (6 Cr App R (S) 444). Here, the defendant pleaded to one count of living on immoral earnings and to aiding and abetting buggery and bestiality. The man was able to keep the woman under his control by threatening to expose her prostitution to the Social Services; the woman complied with his demands fearing that her children would be removed from her care. The woman ran away on three occasions; on each occasion the defendant found her and forcibly brought her back. He advertised her services in a contact magazine and forced her to have intercourse with a dog, pictures of which he then sold to pornographic publishers. Prostitute women are vulnerable to male violence (Jaget 1980: 124; Ohse 1984: 34; Roberts 1986: 81; Edwards 1993a), have died at their hands (Edwards 1991a) and are frequently victims of assault, rape and buggery (see *Wallace* (1990) 27 July unreported; *Wilmot* (1990) 89 Cr App R 341; *Cannan* [1990] Crim LR 869; *Attorney General's Reference No. 12 of 1992* (1993) 14 Cr App R (S) 233; see also Barnard 1993; Edwards 1993a, 1993b).

Part of the struggle of feminists engaged in the arena of prostitution involves efforts to deconstruct and reconstruct prostitution within the domain of the violent rather than the domain of the sexual; this has involved resisting efforts to legitimate prostitution. One of the more visible forms of legitimation has been through state legalization. Evelina Giobbe of WHISPER argues: 'Dismantling the institution of prostitution is the most formidable task facing contemporary feminism'; this means emphasizing the systematic organization of prostitution, which is at the heart of the problem, instead of reducing prostitution to individual prostitute–client encounters abstracted from the societal power structures of which it is a part. The Coalition Against Trafficking in Women, together with other abolitionist societies including the International Abolitionist Federation, is one of several organizations which are convinced that it is systematic organized abuse which is the heartbeat of prostitution.

This institutionalization and organization is part of the culture and economics of some developing countries. On an international scale prostitution involves the selling of women to business associates, to pimps across the world. Prostitution involves sex tourism (Matsui 1984; Ohse 1984: 10), the British and European businessman's trip to Bangkok advertised in the tabloids, and military prostitution (including the American GIs docking in Pattaya and Olongopo for rest and recreation *en route* from their heroics in defence of Kuwait after the Gulf War). Prostitution extends to the thousands of women trapped in pornography under duress, as in the case of Linda Marchiano (Lovelace). The reality of her enslavement was a very far cry from the sexual freedom depicted by her captors.' Prostitution is manifest in forced labour in many countries and in the selling of women as sex slaves. In each of these expressions the prostitution of women and young girls is frequently legitimated as a viable alternative to poverty.

The feminization of poverty throughout the world provides in part a key to understanding the invincible and enduring nature of prostitution and women's involvement in it, whilst patriarchy explains men's control over and sexual exploitation of women. The case of military prostitution serves as just one example of how Western imperialism, heroism and jingoism disguised the 'other side' of the activities of troops whose use of prostitute women covertly supported the prostitution of poor and powerless women in developing countries. Javate de Dios (1991) exposes prostitution as a form of sexual violence and exploitation manifested against Filipino women through sex tourism, military prostitution, migration, mail order brides and pornography. She argues that forty-six years of American colonization and the continuation of US military bases in the Philippines has served to legitimate prostitution. In fact, as Barry found, the American presence not only legitimated and regulated prostitution. In 1972, women working as prostitutes were openly welcomed onto US bases in Vietnam, where they were known as 'local national guests'. At Longbinh, near Saigon, it was reported that soldiers could take onto the base as a 'local national guest' any of the fifty or sixty girls who waited outside the base (Barry 1981: 72). As a recent survey report on *Women Entertainers in Angeles and Olongopo in the Philippines* (Miralao *et al.* 1990: 1) reveals:

> underlying the bases' flesh trade are the exaggerated notions of manliness embedded in military thinking which encourage the control and use of women . . . whether as wives, reserve labor or as prostitutes to serve military objectives and the needs of men in uniform.

Since prostitution is part of Filipino culture and way of life for many, it is curious that prostitution is a crime against public morals under Filipino law. Women are permitted to register as entertainers, 'casa girls' or bar workers. In most cases this is a front for prostitution. The government, in response to activities it cannot control, turns a blind eye. The clientele of the 'casa girl' so-called in Angeles City is provided by American men from the Clark Air Base, and in Olongopo City the clientele is drawn largely from the American men of Subic Naval Base. After the war against Iraq's Saddam Hussein, thousands upon thousands of American soldiers docked in Pattaya in Thailand and at the Subic base in the Philippines. The *Philippine Standard* (25 March 1991) reported: 'Thousands of American marines and sailors turned Desert Storm into a filipino Fiesta on Sunday night, crowding into bars and night-clubs in a wild celebration of the Gulf War.' The *Philippine Daily Inquirer* (March 1991) reported a different side of the celebrations with the story of Rosario Baluyot, 12 years of age, who died as a child prostitute near the Subic base. One of her paedophile customers was charged and acquitted by the Supreme Court on the ground that there was no prima facie case against him in particular. The question remains, is prostitution sex or exploitation?

A violation of human rights

For those who perceive prostitution as exploitation, it is a violation of human rights. Indeed, many of the United Nations Covenants support the view that prostitution is a violation of human rights. The 1949 Convention of 2 December, entitled 'Suppression of the Traffic in Persons and of the Exploitation of the Prostitution of Others', contains in its preamble the following statement: 'prostitution and the accompanying evil of the traffic in persons for the purpose of prostitution are incompatible with the dignity and worth of the human person and endanger the welfare of the individual, the family and the community' (United Nations 1988: 181). Article 1 (1) defines a trafficker as someone who: 'procures, entices or leads away, for purposes of prostitution, another person, even with the consent of that person', and (2): 'exploits the prostitution of another person, even with the consent of that person'. Article 2 (1) agrees to punish any person who: 'keeps or manages, or knowingly finances or takes part in the financing of, a brothel'; and Article 2 (2) any person who 'knowingly lets or rents a building or other place or any part thereof for the purpose of the prostitution of others' (1988: 182). There are also two other Conventions which have a bearing on this question: the Convention on the Elimination of all forms of Racial Discrimination (1963) (in United Nations 1988: 56), and the Convention on the Elimination of all Forms of Discrimination against Women (CEDAW) (1979) (in United Nations 1988: 112). Both address the violation of human rights and condemn sexual and racial discrimination in all its forms.CEDAW (Article 6) states: 'parties shall take all appropriate measures, including legislation, to suppress all forms of traffic in women and exploitation of prostitution of women' (United Nations 1988: 116).

On 11 February 1981, the European Community passed a resolution on the position of women in the EEC. Article 55 asks the Commission to conduct a systematic inquiry into the purpose of prostitution and to carry out a study of the ways of linking suppression of such activities within and between the member states ('Women of Europe', *Official Journal of the European Community* (Brussels) 1981 no. C59: 89). Prostitution in itself violates women's human rights because prostitution is a violation of Articles 1, 4, 5 and 6 respectively of the Universal Declaration of Human Rights (1948), which declares: 'All human beings are born free and equal in dignity and rights. They are endowed with reason and conscience and should act towards one another in a spirit of brotherhood', and: 'No one shall be held in slavery or servitude', and: 'No one shall be subjected to torture, or to cruel, inhuman or degrading treatment . . . ', and: 'everyone has the right to recognition everywhere as a person before the law' (United Nations 1988: 2).

The Coalition Against Trafficking in Women wishes to take the 1949 Convention further and make some important amendments. The Coalition with UNESCO wishes to see a redrafting of the Convention which takes sexual exploitation as its starting point. Sexual exploitation has been the missing aspect from Conventions since 1949 and is also absent from CEDAW. The Coalition Against

Trafficking in Women spearheaded by Kathleen Barry, along with several of its members, including Evelina Giobbe of WHISPER and Dorchen Liedholt and myself, made representations to the United Nations in Geneva. Together we drafted a new Convention Against Sexual Exploitation, arguing that it is a fundamental human right to be free from sexual exploitation in all its forms. Part of that proposed new Convention is to provide mechanisms and structures which will outlaw the positive promotion of sexual exploitation, and challenge the perpetuation of images of women and children which define them as less than human and thereby facilitate the hatred of these groups. Part of this endeavour is to provide positive programmes in education, work and other economic and supportive structures which will diminish the necessity for prostitution. It is, we believe, a form of discrimination embracing racism and sexism; the existence of systems of prostitution serve to condone and legitimate the discriminatory treatment of women at all levels of society.

As practical action the Coalition called for all states to criminalize illegal activities of prostitutes whilst at the same time strengthening penal measures which seek to control the client, the procurer and the pimp, as defined in Articles 1 and 2 of the 1949 Convention. The solution lies with governments taking responsibility to provide viable alternatives to prostitution (Finstad and Hoigard 1993). This is a struggle against exploitation which must continue so long as prostitution is condoned and legitimated.

Prostitution: sexual freedom, a matter of self-determination

The prostitution inequality/coercion argument is challenged by those who argue that prostitution is primarily a matter of sex and of sexual liberation and of freedom (see Pheterson 1989). Prostitution is about providing a sexual service. Since prostitution is a contract freely entered into, then arguments of exploitation and coercion can be rebutted. This conceptualization of prostitution is one which has found favour amongst liberals and amongst prostitutes and those who own and control the sex industry. It is a view which will ensure the perpetuation of prostitution and its corollaries. The politics are naive and confused *laissez faire ad absurdum*. In 1973, the organization COYOTE was founded in the US and in 1985 was affiliated to the International Committee for

Prostitutes' Rights formed in Amsterdam (Pheterson 1989). The basic principles of the alliance are that prostitute women have basic rights to occupational choice, to sexual self-determination and to work as prostitute women. Their struggle is towards the freeing of prostitution from state control and the recognition of prostitution as a legitimate form of work in exactly the same way as any other form of wage labour is recognized. The denial of self-determination for prostitutes and the right to work as a prostitute are their central causes of concern.

Without a doubt the extension of some rights to prostitute women is to be welcomed. Both lobbies recognize the discriminatory practices against women who are engaged in prostitution solely on the basis of their prostitution. Covert legal regulation has meant that prostitute women have not had the same access to services or resources or legal treatment as victims, especially of sex offenders (see Chambers and Millar 1983, 1986), compared with non-prostitute women, in respect of rights, liberties and freedoms around housing, education, health care, and issues relating to the custody and access to children (see *Re Y* (minors) (1990) Fam Law 223; *Re S* (Minors) 6 April 1989 unreported), and even in the exercise of discretion for suitability for a place on an *in vitro* fertilization programme (see Edwards 1989).

The pro-prostitution lobby wishes to press national governments, the UN Working Group on Contemporary forms of Slavery, the Council of Europe and the European Parliament to acknowledge a new convention for the Suppression of Traffic in Persons which would recognize the right to self-determination of prostitute women. The pro-prostitution lobby calls on the UN to differentiate between prostitution as chosen work and forced prostitution. The Netherlands government has not ratified the 1949 Convention on prostitution, on the basis, as the Dutch government sees it, that where prostitution is freely chosen prostitute women should have the right to self-determination. Similarly, the Turkish government takes the view that prostitution is legitimate work and should only be controlled in order to prevent the spread of venereal diseases.

This way of conceptualizing prostitution has also infected the politico-legal arena. Here the Dutch government supports the move towards legalisation through state control, which will lead to prostitution being ultimately recognized as just another form of paid work. Whilst, quite rightly, the Netherlands government, in common with those of other European countries, wishes to outlaw the traffic in women as domestic workers, cultural entertainers and mail-order brides, it seeks to draw a distinction between the latter as forced prostitution and the prostitution of women on the streets of Sussex Gardens, London, or Amsterdam as free prostitution. However, the Dutch government has taken a strong line on what it considers the traffic in women, and the prosecution of a Dutch trafficker, Jan Schoemann, following the sale of Lisa Mamac to a sex farm in Holland, stands as an example of this commitment.

A human right

The pro-prostitution lobby, which seeks to further legitimate prostitution on the grounds of citizenship rights and privacy, has very much adopted the language of human rights to further its cause. Yet this is curious in the light of Article 1 of the Universal Declaration of Human Rights ('all men are born free and equal in dignity and rights'), and any attempt to turn on its head the concept of self-determination and freedom by arguing for the self-determination of a disempowered group to enjoy other inalienable rights with a view to furthering a form of enslavement must be a contradiction in terms. Article 4 of that Declaration states: 'no one shall be held in slavery or servitude', and Article 5: 'no one shall be subjected to torture, or to cruel, inhuman or degrading treatment'. To propose that prostitute women should also have the right to self-determination which facilitates further prostitution, seems on the contrary to be an abrogation of self-determination, dignity and respect.

The way in which this argument is construed depends on how one sees prostitution; it is without doubt confusing. If self-determination for prostitute women allows them to prostitute (which is the argument advanced by the Netherlands government), such a position facilitates the perpetuation of a condition which involves the sale of a woman's body and results in the objectification and dehumanization of the seller or prostitute, a depressed condition which cannot be altered or improved simply because prostitute women are allowed to prostitute. (In the context of class and revolution Marx predicted the embourgeoisement of the proletariat, the increasing apparent improvement of their condition generating a state of false consciousness.) For Plato in the Happy Slave analogy, the tautology is clear: if slaves are given rights to their own enslavement, does that alter the fundamental existence of their slavery?

The issue of self-determination for the 'free' prostitute centres very much on the right to work and to be taxed. All these issues were raised by Lindi St Clair in her struggles with the inspector of taxes. The case of *Aken* raises the issue of whether prostitution is lawful and thus should be as subject to taxation as any other activity. In Europe many prostitute women are seeking to have their activities validated by being taxed like any other profession. The courts in England considered this matter too, albeit not at the instigation of the would be taxpayer but at the instigation of the Inland Revenue. In *Inland Revenue Commissioners* v. *Aken* [1990] (1 WLR 1374), Ms Aken had practised as a prostitute for many years. The Inland Revenue became aware of her income following a television programme about her and the inspector raised assessments under Schedule D (Case 1) for the year 1973–4 on income described as 'professional fees', and for the years 1974–5 to 1980–1 on income described as 'profits of prostitution'. She gave notice of appeal against these assessments but subsequently reached an agreement with the Inland Revenue as to the amount due, although she did not pay the agreed sum. The Inland Revenue issued proceedings against her to recover the tax owed, but the court refused to enter the judgment for the Inland Revenue. The Inland Revenue appealed on the basis that the matter of whether tax should be paid had already been determined in law. She appealed and her appeal was dismissed on the grounds that prostitution was a trade. In *R* v. *Register of Companies ex parte Attorney General* [1991] (BCLC, 476), the court quashed a decision to register Lindi St Clair's (Personal Services Ltd) as a registered company. The Attorney-General applied to quash the incorporation and registration by the Registrar of Companies on 18 December 1979, of Lindi St Clair (Personal Services Ltd) as a registered company under the provisions of the Companies Act 1948 to 1976. The grounds of the application were these. In certifying the incorporation of a company, and in registering the same, the Registrar of Companies acted *ultra vires*, or misdirected himself, so in 1980 it was quashed as the object of the company was to carry on the business of prostitution which, for this purpose, was unlawful. The paradox or conundrum persists: earnings from prostitution are taxable but the British government will not condone prostitution as a lawful trade for the purposes of registration.

THE INCOMING 'SEX INDUSTRY' TIDE OF EUROPE

Whatever the debates and whatever the decisions in Europe, already in the sex industry arena domestic legislation has been compelled to toe the European line. Some countries in Europe have demonstrated an approach to prostitution which favours legalization through a measure of state control. Some European countries have also taken a view which firmly regards prostitution as part of the province of sexuality and therefore a matter of individual freedom and individual choice. A distinction has been made in most European countries between free prostitution and forced prostitution. The legal result is that streetwalking has been decriminalized, so that prostitutes can solicit freely between certain restricted hours in specified areas and are registered and required to bring clients back to the state-regulated brothels in the vicinity. At the same time forced prostitution in the form of pimping and procuring is criminalized and harsh penalties apply.

Nevertheless, as we become increasingly influenced by EC law, there is a concern that their laws will become ours, and in a Europe that perceives prostitution as part of a sex and leisure industry, it may become increasingly difficult to argue that prostitution is part of an industry of exploitation and abuse and one which must be regulated.

How far will UK domestic laws and policy be able, or consider it desirable, to resist the consciousness of the community? Community law has already begun to have its impact and its authority was upheld in *Conegate Ltd* v. *HM Customs and Excise* ([1987] QB 254; [1986] 1 CMLR 739), where it was held that following the EEC Treaty, Article 36, goods lawfully made or sold in the UK can also be imported provided they are of EEC origin. In *Conegate* the haul consisted of inflatable dolls imported from Germany, complete with pubic hair, oral, vaginal and anal orifices. The judgment in *Conegate* has had wider implications for the importation of other pornographic materials into Britain.

Again, EC law has deliberated on the provision of sexual commodities. This freedom to provide services (Articles 58–66) is subject to derogation on the grounds of 'public policy, public security or public health'. In the case of the provision of sex shops, the EC deemed that it had no control in deciding whether sex shops should be established and could not override domestic discretion pertaining to the Local Government Act 1982 (see *Sheptonhurst Ltd* v. *Newham Borough Council* [1991] CMLR 463; *Quietlynn Ltd and Another* v. *Southend Borough Council* [1990] 3 All ER 207; [1990] 3 CMLR 55; [1990] 2 QB 19; *Portsmouth City Council* v. *Brian James Richards* [1989] 1 CMLR 673). Under Article 177 preliminary ruling procedure, respecting regulation of trade imports, the court was called on to assess validity under Community law of the Local Government (Miscellaneous Provisions) Act 1982. The court ruled that Article 30 of the Treaty should be construed as meaning that national provisions prohibiting the sale of lawful sex articles from unlicensed sex establishments do not constitute a measure having an effect equivalent to a quantitative restriction on imports (at 67 the Court Sixth Chamber). In *R* v. *London Borough of Newham ex parte Sheptonhurst* 4 March 1992 LEXIS, *Sheptonhurst Ltd* made an application for judicial review of the decision of the London Borough of Newham against their decision not to grant a sex shop licence; the history of the application goes back to 1984. The application was dismissed. Although, halfway through, the decision on the Shops Act and Sunday trading had been referred to the EC, and was found to be contrary to Art. 2, 30 of the Treaty of Rome, judicial review was halted as it was decided that it was a matter for the EC. The EC found in favour of Newham and referred the case back to the High Court in the UK, with the direction that the case should not have been referred in the first place.

We have, however, so far been able to prohibit transmissions of programmes from Red Hot Dutch, as a result of the public policy commitment to child protection in accordance with Article 22 of the EC Directive on Broadcasting, which ratified the granting of an injunction in April 1993 (*R.* v. *Secretary of State for the National Heritage, ex parte Continental Television BVio and others*, Queen's Bench Division CO/837/93, 23 April 1993, LEXIS, Enggen, whereas appeal by Continental Television against the refusal of the Divisional Court to grant an interlocutory injunction against the Secretary of State for the National Heritage was dismissed), thereby preventing the sale of the equipment necessary for reception of the satellite station transmitting Red Hot Dutch. This was achieved notwithstanding Mr Pannick's argument (for the appellant) that the hours of transmission precluded viewing by minors. Lord Justices Glidewell, Kennedy and Hirst, were of the view that many of the subscribers would record the output because of the time at which it was transmitted, thereby increasing the opportunity for access by minors. Article 22 of the EC Directive on Broadcasting 89/552/EEC dated October 1989 provides that:

> Member states shall take appropriate measures to ensure that television broadcasts by broadcasters under their jurisdiction do not include programmes which might seriously impair the physical, mental, or moral development of minors, in particular those that involve pornography or gratuitous violence. The provision shall extend to other programmes which are likely to impair the physical, mental or moral development of minors, except where it is ensured, by selecting the time of the broadcast or by any technical measure, that minors in the area of transmission will not normally hear or see such broadcasts.

The primary responsibility for ensuring compliance with this requirement rests on the member state in whose jurisdiction the broadcaster is situated (see also Coleman and McMurtrie 1993).

Looking to the EEC Treaty, there are several articles relating to the movement of workers and the rights of residence and of establishment; these articles have implications for the status of all workers in Europe as well as those in the 'sex industry'. The question arises now passport restrictions have been removed etc., whether such decisions will influence workers coming to seek work in the UK 'sex industry' from Europe. The judgments in the *Adoui* and *Roux* cases are of relevance here, since they indicate that, in respect of the regulation of prostitution, we may continue with existing laws which would not be in breach of any EC law on the grounds of 'public policy'. In *Rezguia Adoui and Dominique* v. *Belgian State* ECJ [1982] (3 CMLR 631, 18 May 1982), two French women were expelled from Belgium on the grounds of 'public policy' following their suspected prostitution, although prostitution was not unlawful in Belgium. Miss Adoui applied for a residence permit, which was refused on the grounds that her personal conduct was not approved of as she worked in a bar with waitresses suspected of prostitution. She left and returned one month later summonsing the Belgian State to grant interlocutory relief that she had been the victim of unlawful acts. Miss Cornuaille similarly applied for residence; she too was suspected of prostitution. Her presence in the Netherlands was said to be detrimental to public policy. The court held:

> the public policy provisions in Articles 48 and 56 EEC do not permit a member state to expel a national of another member state (or refuse him access) on the grounds of personal conduct, if such conduct on the part of the local nationals does not give rise to repressive measures or other genuine and effective measures intended to combat such conduct.
>
> (*Regina* v. *Bouchereau* [1977] 2 CMLR 800 followed (at 631)

The Court interpreted Articles 48 and 56 of the EEC Treaty and Articles 6 and 9 of Directive 64/221. The Court ruled: (1) That a member state may not, by virtue of the reservation relating to public policy contained in Articles 48 and 56 of the Treaty, expel a national of another member state from its territory or refuse him access to its territory by reason of conduct which, when attributable to the former state's own nationals, does not give rise to repressive measures or other genuine and effective measures intended to combat such conduct; (2) Circumstances not related to the specific case may not be relied upon.

These cases raise the question of the limits within which member states may, in the light of Community law, adopt individual measures deporting or expelling nationals of other member states who enjoy the benefit of the freedom of movement for workers or the right of establishment (*supra* at 640). In respect of public policy national authorities have been allowed some discretion but not to apply this in an arbitrary manner (*supra* 661): 'Although that difference of treatment, which bears upon the nature of the measures available not to be exercised in an arbitrary manner.' In the case of *Danielle Roux*, a french *fille de joie* who had been a street prostitute in Belgium since 1988, on her arrival in Belgium she applied for a residence permit giving her profession as a waitress. When the authorities discovered the real nature of her work they refused to grant her a work permit, justifying their decision on the grounds that her work 'was not in conformity with the social legislation in force'. In April 1989, Roux took the Belgium state to court challenging its action before the tribunal of the first instance in Liège; the court was unable to rule and referred the case to the European Court in Luxembourg. Under the Treaty of Rome citizens of one country have the right to live in another country, the only condition being that they are pursuing an economic activity; non-conformity with state social legislation is not a reason for denying right of residence. In February 1991, the Court of Justice of the European Communities handed down a judgment in her favour (see *Observer* 10 February 1991; *Official Journal of the European Communities* 5 March 1991).

These several cases relate to free trade of 'sexual' commodities, the right of residence and the right to work for female prostitutes. Whilst 'public policy' may prevail, given that the approach to prostitution in Europe is very different to our own, even if we may not be legally required to bring ourselves into line with Europe, in time we may be forced to do so politically. This will very much depend on how the prostitution debate is defined and articulated in the years ahead, whether as forced or free, a matter of privacy or exploitation, an abrogation of human rights and equality or a human right to be fought for. It is clear, however, that prostitution is regarded as a legitimate dimension of a legitimate industry, the sex industry. There are mighty forces which seek to promote the idea that prostitution is sexual freedom and that those who engage in it do so from personal choice. At the heart of the direction to be taken lies the dichotomy of whether prostitution is a matter of sexual choice, preference and self-determination or part of an institution of exploitation and degradation of women. Those who argue that the latter is the truth will find their voice eclipsed by the mega power of the pornography industry, which continues to sell the lie that prostitution is sex and is a matter of choice. 'You cannot be free if you are contained within a fiction' (Beck, cited in Dworkin 1989). The only people who are free are those perpetuating this fiction, the commercial pimps who print and communicate the lie that prostitution is freedom and the nation states which benefit from the taxes and fines imposed on these women.

Chapter 4

Campaigning for legal change

English Collective of Prostitutes

In 1975 the English Collective of Prostitutes (ECP) came together as an autonomous organization of prostitute women within the International Wages for Housework Campaign. With our sister organization, the US PROStitutes Collective, we form the International Prostitutes Collective – a network of women, Black/of colour and white, of different nationalities and backgrounds, working at various levels of the sex industry. We campaign for the abolition of the prostitution laws which punish women for refusing to be poor and/or financially dependent on men; for human, legal, economic and civil rights for prostitute women; and for higher welfare benefits and wages, student grants, housing and other resources so that no woman, child or man is forced by poverty into sex with anyone.

FOR PROSTITUTES AGAINST PROSTITUTION

When we began, the fight for prostitute women to be acknowledged as part of the women's movement for financial independence and control over our own bodies, and part of the working-class movement for more money and less work, was completely new. It is still controversial. Most of women's liberation was hostile to prostitute women on the grounds that exchanging sex for money was uniquely degrading. They said it encouraged rape by leading men to believe that all women are available, conveniently forgetting that men already thought that. The sex industry is not the only industry which is male-dominated and degrades women, but it is an industry where the workers are illegal and can least defend publicly their right to their jobs and take stands against their employers. We argued that for some women to get paid for what all women are expected to do for free is a source of power for all women to refuse the free sex they don't want.

In 1975, the Wages for Housework Campaign was the only women's organization to come out in support of prostitute women.

> All work is prostitution, whether we work for money or room and board. All women are prostitutes, whether we fuck for money, wait on tables, pack biscuits, type letters, drive lorries, bear children, teach in schools, or work in the coal mines, we are forced to sell our bodies and minds. Our whole lives are stolen from us by work.
>
> . . . all women benefit from prostitutes' successful attempts to receive cash for sexual work, because the cash makes it clear that women are working when we are fucking, dressing up, being nice, putting on make-up, whenever we relate to men. . . . The prostitute, lesbian or 'straight', refuses the unlimited emotional and sexual work (and laundry) that normally accompany relations with men, in favour of a cash demand.
>
> (Power of Women Collective 1975)

Since prostitute women are illegal workers who, most of the time, cannot afford to come out publicly (often not even to family or friends), the ECP called on a non-prostitute woman, Selma James, housewife, mother and founder of the Campaign, to be its first public spokeswoman. Not only was she willing to be trained by prostitute women, she also trained the women in the ECP: her experience as a long-standing organizer in the Black and women's movements helped shape the ECP and developed everyone's skills and confidence.

As more women were able to speak for themselves, we developed a policy of not revealing who was and who wasn't on the game. We wanted our members, illegal working women, to be able to speak out without having to come out. We were determined to choose our spokeswomen on the basis of their ability to represent and be accountable to the prostitute women's movement rather than on their ability to 'come out'.

GUILTY UNTIL PROVEN INNOCENT

Although prostitution *per se* is not illegal in Britain, it is almost impossible for a woman to work as a prostitute without breaking the law.

The 1959 Street Offences Act makes it illegal for a 'common prostitute' – not just any woman – to loiter or solicit for prostitution. This labelling of women as 'common prostitutes' is accomplished by two police cautions before going to court; it denies prostitute women the fundamental right under the law that a defendant is innocent until proven guilty. Unlike others, who are not supposed to be tried on the basis of past convictions, a prostitute woman is judged first of all on her record – not the evidence against her, but the cautions which stamp and condemn her. Her guilt, never having been established, will be confirmed at her first trial and will then 'prove' her further guilt. This presumption of guilt is the basis of every arrest and conviction of prostitute women.

Through our national network we have collected evidence of arbitrary cautions, including retrospective cautions given during arrest: 'We saw you last Friday with a punter, count that as a caution.' Cautions can result in putting women on the game. A Birmingham woman who was cautioned after coming out of a children's home decided that since she now had a record she 'may as well get something for it'.

Most prostitute women do not complain about being arrested when they are breaking the law. What they object to is sexist and – if they are not white and English – racist police behaviour, false arrests, insults, threats and violence, double standards, and demands for free sexual services or for information on other women or clients as a condition of not being arrested. Women have been arrested and handcuffed when not working with the excuse that 'if a punter came up they wouldn't turn him down'. Other women have been arrested coming out of their homes, going to the shops or sitting in their car. One woman was in her slippers! At the police station women are often refused the right to a phone call, access to a solicitor, and in some cases bail, even though the offence for which they are being arrested is no longer prisonable and they have never failed to turn up in court. One woman, after winning six 'not guilty' pleas, took the police to court for harassment and won – she had been arrested 48 times in 52 days.

Magistrates' widespread bias against sex workers ensures that most women plead guilty even when they are not, and that many women end up in jail for an offence which is no longer prisonable because they can't afford to pay their fines. Even under the unit fine system, which was supposed to guarantee that everyone was fined according to their means, some magistrates took into account future earnings from prostitution: they set the fine according to how 'young and pretty' the woman was, fining her more if they thought she could make more money.

Women who work indoors are also criminalized: if they share premises with even one other woman they can be arrested for brothel-keeping; massage parlours, escort agencies, etc., are often raided and those who run them charged with running a brothel.

Such criminalization creates the much vilified red-light areas as one way in which prostitute women and clients can meet without paying middlemen.

Criminalized and stigmatized by the law, sex workers are denied basic civil rights. They are forced underground for fear of losing custody of children, housing or second job, being deported, ostracized by families and friends, and denied the right to a family life other people take for granted because anyone who associates with a prostitute can be accused of being a prostitute herself or even a pimp. The law makes no distinction between real pimps and men who are husbands, boyfriends or sons; any man who lives wholly or partly on the earnings of prostitution can be charged with pimping – accepting part of the rent money or money for bills, or even a drink, from a prostitute can be enough.

LEGAL DEFENCE

In April 1982 we initiated Legal Action for Women (LAW), a grassroots legal service for all women, in response to prostitute women's needs for advice and support. LAW, and our rights sheet, 'A Guide to the Rules of the Game – A–Z for Working Girls', issued in 1981 and distributed in red-light areas all over the country, launched a movement of women pleading not guilty to prostitution offences in court.

For the following few months the already crowded King's Cross Women's Centre where we were based was busy with all kinds of women. Local prostitute women came in for help with custody cases – children taken into care because their mothers were considered unfit; evictions and other housing matters; and the wide range of legal problems they shared with other women. Many sex workers wanted advice and support with pleading not guilty when arrested illegally – whilst doing their shopping, collecting their children or waiting at a bus stop. LAW found (and in some cases trained) lawyers who were ready to defend women in the way they wanted to be defended, and women started winning their cases in court. One young Black woman with two children told the court she was paying an exorbitant rent and said: 'When I don't have to pay that rent, I won't be a prostitute.' She was found not guilty.

We reported in our newsletter:

> After we won a couple of cases the police got worried. They began keeping an eye on the Centre and picking on the women who used it, many of whom were Black, and women who worked for themselves, without pimps. On several occasions we had to get lawyers to accompany women to the station to prevent the police who were sitting outside the Centre arresting them as they left. They arrested a girl's boyfriend because she was pleading not guilty. They threatened the girl's best friend with taking her kid away, and even told her mother up North what she was doing – just to break up her family.
>
> At the same time the police refused to arrest pimps and rapists when we reported them. One of the girls, who was threatened by a pimp that he would break her ribs if she didn't hand over her money, was told when she reported it to the police that they couldn't do anything until her ribs were broken. A non-prostitute woman was raped in the area. When she reported it, the police accused her of being a prostitute and arrested her boyfriend for pimping because he's Black. They gave her such a grilling at the police station that she withdrew her complaint.
>
> (*Network* 1983)

THE FIRST SANCTUARY

We had to do something to protect ourselves and our families. We knew that in 1975, prostitutes in France went on strike and occupied churches all over the country to protest against police harassment. Following their example, on 17 November 1982, we walked into the Holy Cross Church in King's Cross, with the support of Black Women for Wages for Housework and Women Against Rape. Our banner outside the church read 'Mothers Need Money. End Police Illegality and Racism in King's Cross.' We were demanding that others take a stand with prostitute women in defence of sex workers' legal and civil rights. The occupation lasted twelve days and was a major success – it put the policing of prostitute women on the political agenda. In *Hookers in the House of the Lord*, Selma James writes:

> One Black woman . . . spelled out that the prostitution laws are to young Black women what the 'sus' laws are to young Black men. This was a real breakthrough for us. After years of work, we could begin to see the illegality and racism of the police against hookers being lifted out of the exotic, even the erotic, where it could be dismissed and ridiculed; and onto the deadly serious terrain we share with others who are up against the law.
>
> It also started to break down the barriers between prostitute women and other working-class people. We were on major national television news almost every day, and gathered a lot of support from a wide range of individuals and organizations. Working women from other areas, local residents, members of the church, Black and immigrant women's organizations, women from Greenham and Molesworth peace camps, lesbian women, gay and heterosexual men, brought food and blankets, cooked, babysat for our children and donated money towards the cost of heating the Church.
>
> (James 1984)

That first night in the Church we issued the following press release:

> We are here to demand:
>
> 1. An end to illegal arrests of prostitutes;
> 2. An end to police threats, blackmail, harassment and racism;
> 3. Hands off our children – we don't want our kids in care;
> 4. An end to arrests of boyfriends, husbands, sons;
> 5. Arrest rapists and pimps instead;
> 6. Immediate protection, welfare, housing for women who want to get off the game.

And we asked to see councillors, MPs and representatives of the Home Office.

Several MPs and councillors came to meet with us to see what we wanted. Every day some of us went out to different red-light areas to let the girls outside know what was happening inside. Some women who were still working in Argyle Square wore masks and badges in solidarity with the occupation. News of the occupation travelled fast and prostitute women in other countries organized support. We received telegrams from Italy, Germany, Canada and the United States.

The police were furious. Although arrests dropped dramatically during the occupation because of the glare of publicity, we knew there would be retaliatory arrests as soon as we left the church. We asked the council to appoint a monitor to watch the police to prevent illegal arrests and victimization. We wanted a comparison of arrest figures with and without a monitor to substantiate our claim of police illegality. We won a monitor and firm promises that our other demands would also be met, such as meetings with MPs and the police and someone in the Council Housing Department to refer for help any woman who wanted to leave prostitution – so we left the church.

The monitor's report was released on 20 January 1983. It did not mention the occupation, and anyone reading it now would never suspect that her job was the product of our struggle. Making us invisible was not an oversight. It was an attempt to hijack the legal and other services prostitute women had created. The report had no comparative figures for police arrests. After all that had happened, our claims of police illegality and racism had been sidestepped. We called the report a 'careerist charter' because it signalled to anyone hoping to make a career out of prostitute women's demands that they need not refer proposals about prostitutes and prostitution to prostitutes. Feminists making a career off prostitution has become a new branch of the sex industry and is as much pimping off women as men have ever done.

Twelve years later in King's Cross, politicians and the police are still calling for more policing to 'clean the streets' of prostitute women. Yet for many years the only 'service' that has been poured into the area has been policing – community services and resources have all been cut. The police have been using prostitution to lobby local residents for an increased budget. At the same time councillors are targeting prostitute women in order to be seen to be 'doing something' about the problems of run down inner-city areas and to divert attention from the devastation caused by the Tory cuts which they have implemented.

KERB-CRAWLING LEGISLATION – A NEW 'SUS' LAW

Police illegality has been further encouraged by legislation against kerb-crawling (men soliciting women for sexual purposes), which was introduced in 1985 in the name of bringing equality to prostitute women by arresting their clients, and safety to other women by making it illegal for men to accost them. It has equalized women down by taking away some of the rights men had which women were fighting to get: instead of prostitute women not being arrested for soliciting men, men are being arrested for soliciting women.

In 1984, we initiated the Campaign Against Kerb-Crawling Legislation (CAKCL) – a coalition of anti-rape, Black and civil rights organizations, AIDS prevention groups, lawyers, probation officers and Labour Party activists. We predicted that the then bill would become a new 'sus' law.[1]

Kerb-crawling legislation has extended to heterosexual men some of the biases the prostitution laws inflict on women and gay men. As with loitering and soliciting, the word of the police is enough to convict men of kerb-crawling. The need for corroboration is purposely left out of the law on the grounds that witnesses would be reluctant to give evidence. Giving evidence is always hard, but it is crucial to establish the truth and protect the rights of defendants. The well-publicized 'miscarriage of justice' cases like the Guildford Four, the Birmingham Six, the Tottenham Three, Judith Ward and Stefan Kiszko have shown the dangers of convictions based solely on police evidence.

Yet the government has announced its intention to amend kerb-crawling legislation 'to remove the need to prove persistence, annoyance or nuisance before a man can be convicted of the offence' (*The Independent* 3 March 1993). This requirement was introduced by the House of Lords as a result of CAKCL's objections and is the only legal restraint against false arrest – without it any street exchange between a woman and a man could be criminalized, especially, but not only, if the woman is a prostitute.

Given well-documented police racism and other discrimination, police are likely to use any new powers against Black, Irish, immigrant and other working-class men they may want to charge for unconnected purposes.

Kerb-crawling legislation is part of the government's drive to 'clean-up' inner city areas of one of the more visible effects of their economic policies – increased prostitution – and to defend the value of some people's property at the expense of the civil rights of others. It has also fuelled prejudice and hostility against prostitute women, making it easier for the police to justify increased surveillance in red-light areas: video recording on high streets and in police vans has become standard, and the government has recently approved a relaxation in planning law to allow a further increase in security cameras on high streets.

Although kerb-crawling legislation is about men, it has resulted in larger numbers of prostitute women being arrested. Women – not men – are the first target. In 1992 in England and Wales, according to Home Office figures, there were 9,459 prosecutions for loitering and soliciting (8,787 convictions); 1,089 prosecutions for kerb-crawling (889 convictions); 89 prosecutions for pimping (23 convictions).

The police are using the discrepancy between the number of women and men arrested to claim they need more powers to arrest the clients. The point, however, is not that more men should be arrested but that neither women nor men should be criminalized for consenting sex.

LEGALIZED PROSTITUTION: ASSEMBLY LINES OF SEX

In Birmingham some councillors have been advocating legalized prostitution in the form of toleration zones. We oppose legalized prostitution, including toleration zones in which prostitute women are 'tolerated' while they continue to face arrest if they work outside the designated areas. In Germany and Nevada, legalized brothels have increased police powers and institutionalized pimping by the state, making it harder for women to keep their earnings or to bargain to determine their working conditions. To avoid arrest, prostitute women in Hamburg must register with the police, have compulsory health checks and carry a health pass. A police record makes it harder for women to leave prostitution.

In Germany's Eros centres, competition is fierce; the rents are high and women have to work longer shifts to keep their rooms and pay the middlemen who run them. Only 12 per cent of prostitute women are estimated to work in the legalized area of Hamburg. Women prefer to work illegally rather than submit to the exploitation of state-run sex factories.

> In Germany, legalized prostitutes pay 56 percent of their earnings in taxes but, unlike other taxpayers, are not eligible for any social benefits. In Austria, prostitutes have to report to the police simply to go on holiday.
>
> (*Guardian* 12 May 1992: 36)

In Nevada, women are segregated, forced to work away from their families for six weeks at a time, and denied the right to refuse clients.

The prostitutes' movement has always opposed legalization. In 1975, prostitute women who occupied churches all over France stated:

> We refuse firmly: the re-opening of brothels, even in their modern and luxurious form of Eros centres; to be civil servants of sex completely without freedom; to be nationalized; to be municipalized.
>
> (Jaget 1980: 19)

In 1979, prostitute women in Southampton and Bristol organized against local council proposals for municipal brothels. A Southampton woman spoke for all: 'They would have to bring in the army to get us out of our homes and into their brothels' (James 1984: 184). Neither will such sex ghettoes safeguard the reputation of clients as they would not remove the stigma attached to prostitution.

Who would then benefit from legalized brothels? Lindi St Clair, one of the few prostitute women who openly advocate legalization, is explicit: 'Prostitutes would split their income 50/50 with the Madam. . . . A brothel with 10 prostitutes each earning £1000 pw would turn over £520,000 pa.'[2] The brothels of Madam St Clair would increase government control over prostitute women and tax revenue derived from them, and divide sex workers further between those who get licences and those who don't. Women and young people who are not well-heeled or old enough to set themselves up 'in business' would be fodder for the new sex managers. This two-tier system is already operating. In Amsterdam under the new licensing system immigrant women are prevented from working in the windows in the red-light area.

Toleration zones would not ensure the safety of prostitute women. Zones like those proposed for Birmingham are in non-residential areas where women don't have the protection of other people being out on the streets. The Birmingham police have said that they would want increased powers to arrest women who refuse to work there. In Utrecht women have complained about being arrested going back and forth from the toleration zones, and about the police 'washing their hands of the area' and refusing to protect them from violence.

WHEN PROSTITUTE WOMEN AREN'T SAFE NO WOMAN IS SAFE

The prostitution laws divide women between those of us who are considered 'good' and 'respectable' and those of us who are considered 'bad' and 'loose' for refusing poverty by working in the sex industry.

By signalling to men that prostitute women are criminals and that violence against them will be dealt with leniently, the prostitution laws make it more dangerous for women to work. Sex workers cannot rely on the protection of the police and the courts against pimps, rapists and other violent men. Attacks which women report to the police are often dismissed as 'part of the job'. Even when the police response is not hostile or unsympathetic it lacks the coordinated approach of anti-prostitution crackdowns.

In 1981 we picketed the High Court throughout the trial of the Yorkshire Ripper, a serial murderer who killed thirteen women and attacked many others. As in the case of the Green River murders in Canada and Seattle, and the Los Angeles South Side murders, the police used the prostitution laws as an excuse to do nothing, labelling as prostitutes the murdered women, who were in any case Black and/or too poor to matter. The police only took the murders seriously after a relatively better off 'respectable' woman was killed. Many more women died as a result, prostitute and non-prostitute alike.

Kerb-crawling legislation has added to prostitute and other women's vulnerability to violence by: forcing working women further underground; curtailing the time available for prostitute women to 'sus out' clients, nervous about arrest before going with them; committing more police time and resources to prostitution rather than rape and other violent crimes.

Despite requests from the ECP and Women Against Rape (WAR), the police have refused to say how much of their time and resources go into prostitution and how much into violent crimes. They justify their 'clean-ups' by saying that they have to respond to local public demand. Yet, Black communities have long been pressing for the arrest and conviction of those responsible for racist attacks. The police have done little or nothing. They decide which 'public' they will respond to, and which they'll ignore.

Women in Bristol, Leicester, Manchester, Swindon, Walsall and the London red-light areas of Balham, Bayswater and King's Cross, have confirmed an increase in violence which the police have done little or nothing about. A typical example is that of a Black woman who was almost strangled: when the police arrived they ignored the guilty man sitting across the road and arrested her instead. In King's Cross, special police squads regularly arrest hundreds of women and men in a combined effort to 'clean up' the area, while failing to act to solve murders and rapes.

This is happening right now in the Midlands where at least seven women – four of whom have been labelled as prostitutes by the police – have been murdered this year in similar circumstances. Instead of protecting women the police have stepped up the arrest of working women and clients. These serial murders are quickly becoming another Ripper case.

We have been urging MPs, Police Committees, Community Affairs Committees in areas where the murders have taken place, the All-Party Parliamentary Group on Prostitution, and Church leaders to support our call for action which targets the murderer/s, not prostitute women and clients, including a temporary amnesty for prostitution offences to enable anyone to come forward with information without fear of arrest. The police have refused.

The police are not alone in dismissing violence against sex workers. In 1981, we protested the verdict in the case of Peter Swindell, a policeman accused of killing Pat Malone, a lesbian prostitute woman. Although he admitted dismembering her body he was found not guilty of manslaughter. We wrote: 'were the situation reversed and a lesbian prostitute was accused of killing a policeman she would have been convicted, not of manslaughter, but of murder, and sentenced to life'.[3]

In 1981 we picketed the Old Bailey throughout the trial of the Yorkshire Ripper, Peter Sutcliffe, in protest against the prosecuting Attorney General, Sir Michael Havers, saying of the Ripper victims that: 'some were prostitutes, but perhaps the saddest part of this case is that some were not. The last six attacks were on totally respectable women.'

Another example is the case of PC Anderson, a policeman convicted of raping a young Black single mother while on duty. He used the police computer to check if she had any convictions for prostitution and threatened her with arrest for soliciting is she dared report the rape. The jury found him guilty but he was later released on appeal on the basis of a technicality: the appeal judge said not enough weight had been given to his 'good' character (*The Voice* 10 July 1980: 1).

Recent media coverage has highlighted how the Crown Prosecution Service (CPS) often drops cases where the victim is a prostitute or the criminal a police officer. In October 1991, we asked the CPS if the resignation of the former DPP, Sir Allan Green, stopped for kerb-crawling in King's Cross, signalled the end of prosecutions against police officers who had broken the law in far more serious and vicious ways than Sir Allan may have, and whether the police were issuing a warning of what may happen to others if such prosecutions continued. Sir Allan had initiated several prosecutions against senior police officers involved in 'miscarriage of justice' cases.

> Prosecutions seems to have less to do with evidence than with the status of the accused: a common feature of 'miscarriages of justice' is precisely how little evidence there was against the defendant; another feature is that the defendants were Black, Irish and/or working class, young, and that many had a record for petty crimes. Police officers, on the other hand, are rarely prosecuted and, when they are, almost always have the backing of the judiciary.
>
> (*Guardian* 25 May 1992)

A number of prosecutions have been dropped since against officers and against rapists.

Together with WAR, we are supporting two prostitute women who were violently raped while working for an escort agency. In spite of much clear evidence the CPS decided not to prosecute. The women have launched a private prosecution. Women Against Rape has been challenging CPS decisions not to prosecute on a number of other cases involving Black women, women with disabilities and children.

More women are realizing that their lives and safety are tied up with the lives and safety of their illegal sisters. In December 1989, the ECP and WAR supported a woman whose ex-husband, Victor Powell, was being sentenced for the rape of a prostitute woman. We held a vigil outside the court to highlight the vulnerability that prostitute women and wives share at the hands of the law, the police and the courts. Powell had repeatedly attacked his wife and broken injunctions to stay away from her. The fact that rape in marriage was not illegal until October 1991 has affected whether the police treat all domestic violence and rape seriously. Powell was never prosecuted for attacking his wife. She and her children were put at risk by court delays and by police refusing to act before receiving official notification – usually two days after the court order.

He also had previous convictions for raping another two prostitute women. In this case the woman was held prisoner, raped and assaulted in his home. Drinking heavily, he eventually fell asleep and she managed to call the police. They took 45 minutes to arrive.

Contradicting stereotypes that wives and prostitutes are inevitable sworn enemies, Powell's ex-wife, who suffered years of violence at his hands, and the prostitute woman he raped, met at the trial and became friends. Each sees the guilty verdict and the life sentence passed for the rape as a protection. It is a victory or all women when the rape of prostitute women is recognized as rape.

RESISTING THE VIRUS OF REPRESSION

As soon as AIDS was labelled as a 'sexually transmitted disease', sex workers knew another witch-hunt was in the making. Gay men, prostitute women, Black and immigrant people were blamed for 'spreading AIDS': physically attacked, deported or stopped at the border, forced to have HIV tests, evicted, sacked, imprisoned, mothers who were HIV positive were threatened with losing custody of their children.

In April 1992 the King's Cross police were reported in the press alleging that 'of the 50 hard-core regulars who work the streets around the station . . . three out of four have the virus (*Sunday Express* 29 April 1992). When we asked for the source of such 'information' they told us that it came from a police survey. A copy of it revealed that it asked no question about either HIV or AIDS. What the survey does address, however, is the lack of police response to violence reported by prostitute women. This, of course, was not publicized. The police have never apologized for or corrected their scaremongering disinformation.

In San Francisco, the US PROStitutes Collective is spearheading opposition to City Council proposals to declare a public health emergency and legalize prostitution. Legalization would extend mandatory HIV testing to all prostitute women. This is despite evidence showing that prostitute women do not have higher rates of HIV than other women, and that men do not get

AIDS through contact with women – prostitute or not. In New York, only 12 out of 29,992 men could claim to have got AIDS from 'sex with women at risk'.[4] Segregating sex workers from the rest of the community is little short of opening internment camps, a dangerous precedent which could be used against anyone labelled 'high risk' for HIV or AIDS or accused of 'spreading disease'.

The AIDS crisis has not invented 'safer sex' – prostitute women have traditionally used condoms as a barrier against VD and unwanted pregnancies. Some women have been ready to refuse offers of up to four times the going rate for sex without a condom. But sex workers' efforts to implement 'safer sex' have been obstructed by the police and court policy of using possession of condoms as evidence of loitering or soliciting. We succeeded in changing this policy. After two years of campaigning to publicize the issue and mobilize public opinion, the Metropolitan police gave in. On 26 July 1993 they wrote back:

> it is not our policy to include in evidence that a woman was found in possession of condoms and we recognise that to do so would conflict with government initiatives that promote safe sexual practices.

In our book *Prostitute Women and AIDS: Resisting the Virus of Repression* we have outlined some of the other victories of the movement against AIDS.

> In spite of the panic and misinformation which keeps pouring out, the movement against AIDS has challenged the AIDS industry: questioning the funding priorities of governments and attacking the profiteering of drug companies; pressing for welfare benefits and other resources for people with AIDS; increasing the visibility of gay men and, to a lesser extent, sex workers and lesbian women; defending the civil rights of people with AIDS or who test HIV positive; establishing that whatever our 'lifestyle', no one is 'asking for AIDS'; refusing to take the blame for AIDS while taking the responsibility for fighting it; surviving in spite of all the medical predictions and telling others how you did it . . .
>
> (Lopez-Jones 1992: 14)

Increasingly people are spelling out the extent to which drug companies dictate AIDS policies and the responsibility of AIDS organizations which have backed such policies at the expense of people's health.

With our sister organization, Black Women for Wages for Housework, we are campaigning to stop the PENTA 1 Trial in which HIV-positive babies and children with no symptoms of AIDS are being given the highly toxic drug AZT. This is despite the result of the Concorde study which established that AZT is of no benefit to HIV-positive adults. Many of the children in the Trial are of African descent. One mother we spoke to said she had not been told that AZT was chemotherapy. She had been reluctant to cooperate, but feared she would be deported if she refused. We took part in a picket outside Great Ormond Street Children's Hospital, one of the main hospitals participating in the Trial, and in a delegation to the Medical Research Council which is funding the Trial. The delegation called by the Standing Committee Against AZT Malpractice (SCAM) of which we are members, presented a document to the MRC stating that Wellcome, the manufacturers of AZT, are in a position to exercise substantial influence in the MRC and in the PENTA 1 Trial through funding, personnal and control over information, and that the PENTA Trial is racist.

We have also publicized evidence refuting the official claim of an African AIDS epidemic. Some prostitute women on the Ivory Coast and in other African countries may be HIV positive but there is little evidence that they are dying or that those who are are dying of AIDS. Black Women for Wages for Housework has spelled out the implications of economic and social policies based on the AIDS scare.

> Investment in the myth of AIDS in Africa enables disinvestment in overcoming genuinely epidemic diseases of poverty such as malnutrition, malaria and tuberculosis. This is having genocidal consequences.
>
> (*Sunday Times* 14 Nov. 1993)

WOMEN'S POVERTY

It is widely recognized that increased poverty, homelessness and unemployment forced more women and young people on the game. According to government figures the number of people living below the 'poverty line' has gone up from 5 million in 1979 to 13.5 million in 1993. There are now over 80,000 teenagers with no income at all (*The Independent* 5 Nov. 1993).

Government policies such as the Child Support Act are making people even poorer. Referred to as 'the most draconian and Dickensian piece of social legislation for decades' by a Parliamentary Early Day Motion (no. 1313, 3 Feb. 1993), the Act forces single mothers on benefits to authorize the collection of maintenance from 'absent fathers'. All the money the father pays is deducted from the mother's Income Support. Women who refuse to cooperate with the Child Support Agency may have £9.14 deducted from their benefit. With her Income Support substantially reduced or even cut – if the father's maintenance assessment covers it she loses her entitlement to benefit – the mother becomes financially dependent on a man she may not want to be in touch with, who may be violent, or who may not be able to afford the extortionate payments imposed by the Agency. More women and children are being pushed onto the streets to live and to work as a result. A total of 36,500 women have been driven off Income Support in this way – no one knows whether and how they are surviving but for many the choice is between prostitution, destitution, low-waged jobs or other forms of exploitation.

This attack on single mothers' right to financial independence from men and to state support for the work of raising children has gone hand in hand with blaming women for the break-up of the nuclear family, youth crime and other 'social ills'. Many women have had to leave relationships to protect themselves and their children from violence. But instead of being commended for their efforts to protect themselves and their children, they are blamed for the poverty that results.

Women who take the often courageous and difficult decision to go on the game to support their families are similarly blamed for prostitution.

> First of all, it strikes me that it is an act of courage not only to go on the game; not only to confront all of society which says that you're immoral if you go on the game and to confront the law which says you're illegal if you go on the game. It's also an act of courage to hold your head up after you have done something which society refuses to acknowledge as in any way a contribution to that society, and have your dignity intact. And I think that part of the motivation for the prostitution laws is precisely to undermine those of us who are prostitutes and those of us who solve our financial problems in other ways that

> are supposed to demoralise us. We retain our dignity, at least we keep more of our dignity intact than they like. And the powers that be are bloody angry that we are able to survive so well doing things that they said we should not do.
>
> (James 1980)

COUNTING WOMEN'S WORK AND ABOLITION OF THE PROSTITUTION LAWS

The United Nation's figure that women do two-thirds of the world's work for 5 per cent of the income and 1 per cent of the assets spells out the history of prostitution – why women are the sellers and men the buyers. As part of the Wages for Housework Campaign, we are pressing for implementation of the 1985 UN decision to count all women's work – in the home, on the land and in the community – in every country's gross national product. The ECP and US PROS want to ensure that the work of prostitute women, which has been essential to the survival of millions of families, entire communities and even countries, is made visible and acknowledged as the economic contribution to society it really is. Counting women's work strengthens the case for the abolition of the prostitution laws: women should not be criminalized for providing some of what the welfare state doesn't provide.

Counting prostitute women's work unveils the sex work and emotional work all women are forced to do – at home, on the job, on the street – gratifying men's sexual demands and egos with understanding and encouraging smiles, words and acts. Counting all women's work, including sex work, is a strategy for crossing the divide between sex workers and other women. It strengthens all women's case for compensation, in the form of increased benefits, wages, services and other resources, for the poverty and overwork which have been forced on most of us – the economic power to refuse all forms of prostitution.

WINNING PUBLIC SUPPORT

Since we began in 1975 and since the 1982 occupation, we have gathered much support. Increasingly people realize that only the abolition of the prostitution laws can both begin to disentangle consenting sex, which should not be the business of the law, from offences of nuisance, and remove the stigma attached to prostitution.

Abolition would also allow women to work from premises and advertise in contact magazines without being charged with brothel-keeping, thus undermining the need for the much vilified red-light areas.

In June 1992 we took legal action against British Telecom for cutting off the phones of a number of prostitute women who advertise in phone boxes. BT expected to get away with it because the women were prostitutes. But OFTEL, the consumer watchdog for telecommunications, ruled that the phones should be re-connected. Although BT was forced to climb down, many women had already paid a high price for BT's illegality – some women lost their business and had to move out. This is not the only time BT has targeted prostitute women. In July 1992 we defeated a clause in the London Local Authorities Bill, jointly promoted by Westminster Council, British Telecom and the Metropolitan Police, which would have criminalized anyone putting cards in phone boxes. In our evidence to the House of Lords Committee we argued that the Clause would:

> Force more women and young people onto the streets where they will face arrests, violence and persecution . . . increase complaints by 'respectable' residents in red-light areas.[5]

The Lords ruled in our favour and the clause was dropped.

In July 1992, the Mothers' Union stated their opposition to legalization and asked that any legal change should take into account the interests of prostitute women. In April 1993, the Royal College of Nursing passed policy recommendations calling for health services which are 'comprehensive, of high quality, local and open/available at suitable times'; 'the police [to] immediately change their practice of using condoms as evidence of prostitution'; and a review of the law which labels a woman 'a common prostitute without testing the evidence in court', and of 'the policy of fining women and men who prostitute so that they have little choice but to continue to prostitute themselves to pay the fines' (RCN 1993).

In 1994 the Liberal Democrats also passed a policy in support of sex workers' civil rights. The policy makes clear that criminalization makes it more dangerous for prostitute women and men to work and harder to get off the game. It calls for the abolition of the prostitution laws and for three women to be able to work from the same premises. Larger establishments would be subject to health and safety and planning regulations.

The advertising campaign run for us free of charge by Bartle, Bogle and Hegarty (BBH) on the 10th anniversary of our Church Occupation, shows how far public opinion has come since 1975. Four slogans went up on posters all over London. They read:

> No-one screws more prostitutes than the government. In 1990 prostitutes were fined £½ million.
>
> What's the difference between a phone company and a prostitute? One charges 48p per min for sex, the other gets charged in court.
>
> Practising safe sex can get you arrested. Prostitutes are arrested for carrying condoms.
>
> What do you call men who take money from prostitutes? Magistrates.

And under every slogan it said:

> Tell your MP to abolish the prostitution laws.

BBH didn't know whether they would be attacked for supporting prostitute women. The response was overwhelming – all the calls we received, except one, agreed with the posters. The times they are a-changing. Power to the sisters.

Part III

The business of selling sex

Chapter 5

Conspicuous and inconspicuous sex work

The neglect of the ordinary and mundane

Graham Scambler

INTRODUCTION

Popular images and stereotypes of the sex worker or prostitute are concentrated largely, if by no means exclusively, on the street worker, who is typically held to be amoral, conspicuously vulgar and indiscriminate and a lost and hopeless victim of abusers and manipulators.

> When people picture a hooker, they picture a woman with a wig, a lot of make up, high heels, short skirt, and fishnet pantyhose.
> ('Jasmin' 1933: 34)

> It makes me furious when women are portrayed as walking, downtrodden victims. . . . Why are girls always portrayed the way they are in the media? We are portrayed as women who stand on street corners, who wear microscopic miniskirts, who are foul-mouthed junkies, who are violent, with severe psychiatric disorders, and who were abused as kids.
> ('Barbara' 1993: 13)

It is the street worker too who attracts the attention of politicians, the police and other agencies of moral regulation and surveillance. This is not surprising when such a high proportion of off-street or indoor workers are inconspicuous to the point of invisibility. Boyle (1994: 11) may be exaggerating the statistics, but her statement that 'the prostitution trade is akin to an iceberg – nine-tenths of it are hidden – with street girls being the visible tip', is well taken. In this chapter some of the more salient and misleading myths about sex workers are debunked, and both the 'normality' claimed by women like 'Jasmin' and 'Barbara' and the mundane everyday aspects of the sex business brought into clearer focus.

In the opening section it is suggested that popular stereotypes of the sex worker, like all social stereotypes embody predictable types of error, and these are then discussed in terms of 'the whore stigma'. The second section draws on published and other material to comment on the day-to-day form and content of the lives of women committed to the sex industry. In the concluding section some of the ramifications of the results of the process of demythologization and demystification practised here and in other chapters in this volume are addressed.

STEREOTYPES, SEXUALITY AND SOCIETY

Since we all inevitably rely on stereotyping, mere condemnations of stereotyped thinking are less than helpful. In the words of McCall and Simmons (1966: 114):

> all living creatures . . . must employ stereotypes to categorize and deal with the kaleidoscopic flow of events around them. Nor can they wait contemplatively until all the facts are in; they must prejudge the meaning of the whole on the basis of a few signs and must act upon this jot of knowledge.

There is no logical reason why such stereotypes should be erroneous, although they can of course only partially fit individuals. However, insofar a they do err, they err in predictable ways. McCall and Simmons usefully list four such 'types' of error: (1) the inclusion of characteristics that are missing in the majority of cases ('errors of commission'); (2) the exclusion of characteristics that are present in the majority of cases ('errors of omission'); (3) the exaggeration of those characteristics that are most pertinent to the projects of those who stereotype; and (4) the imputation of fixed characteristics when in reality these wax and wane.

If the existence of popular stereotypes of the sex worker seems inevitable then, the *nature* of contemporary stereotypes, their mixture of truth and error, and the types of error they contain, are contingent and of interest and concern. Pheterson's (1993) analysis of the whore stigma is instructive here. She begins with a commentary on dictionary definitions of whore/prostitute worth quoting in full:

> *Whore* means *prostitute*. And a prostitute is a woman who offers to hire her body for indiscriminate sexual intercourse, or so says

> *The Concise Oxford Dictionary*. *Prostitute* is further defined as a verb: to prostitute oneself is to sell one's honour for base gain or to put one's abilities to infamous use. Other dictionaries include men secondarily in the noun definition and specify in the verb definition the *shame* attached to dishonour and the *unworthiness* and *wrongdoing* attached to infamous use. The noun clearly denotes a person, especially a woman, offering heterosexual sex, in particular intercourse, for money; the verb denotes any person's activity, which need not be sexual, put to uncommendable use. Those meanings are likely to conform to popular opinion except that many people collapse the second definition into the first. A prostitute then becomes one who sells her honour by offering to hire her body for base gain or for an unworthy doing, specifically sexual intercourse.
>
> (1993: 39)

As Pheterson points out, many women sex workers would baulk at the reference here to '*indiscriminate* sexual intercourse', regarding the selection of both clients and sexual practices as fundamental rights within the trade, if not ones they are always able to assert. Quite frequently sex work does not involve intercourse: in fact some women engage in regular sex work without ever offering or consenting to either vaginal or anal intercourse. The variety of sexual practices sought and satisfied within the industry, often but not always on women's terms, from quick 'hand jobs' and oral sex to the protracted fulfilment of elaborate fetishes calling for acting rather than explicitly sexual skills, defies easy summary.

Pheterson goes on to provide a useful analysis of the 'dishonour' associated with sex work, considering the ramifications of its *legal*, *social*, *psychological* and *ideological* aspects for sex workers, clients and pimps. The following discussion draws heavily on her work. In relation to *legal dishonour*, she aptly and ironically observes (1993: 43) that women are allowed to give free sex but not to negotiate with a view to payment without defying a host of laws: 'A woman who earns money through sex is defined as selling her honour.' Even in countries like Britain, where prostitution itself is not illegal, many women sex workers, and especially street workers offending against the Street Offences Act of 1959, find it all but impossible in practice to avoid law-breaking and often also find their civil liberties and rights at risk. As 'Julie' angrily explained to McLeod (1982: 116):

> The law gets me down. It says being a prostitute isn't illegal. They can even make you pay tax on it. God forbid! But having said that, 'Okay you can be a prostitute', they then proceed to make it as difficult as possible for you. You can't advertise, no one can let you premises. If you live with someone they can be done for living off immoral earnings. If two of you share a house or flat it's a brothel if you're working from there. If you've got convictions as a common prostitute you can be walking along, say even for a bag of chips, and they can get you.

Families, friends and clients, as well as pimps, are vulnerable too.

Unsurprisingly, Britain's prostitution laws are not applied equally to sex worker and client. No less predictably, attempts to reduce this inequality by penalizing clients – witness the Sexual Offences Act of 1985 which outlawed kerb-crawling – are opposed by sex workers. Pheterson (1993: 44) quotes one sex worker as follows:

> First of all, arresting johns is bad for business. Secondly, it pushes us further underground where we're more vulnerable. And thirdly, it misses the point: we want as much right to sell sex as men have to buy it; we don't want punishment for them – we want *rights for us*.

Nor has such legislation aimed at clients proved effective in Britain or elsewhere.

More assiduous attempts have been made in the past and the present to legislate against third parties like pimps, defined in the Sexual Offences Act of 1956 as persons who profit from the earnings of a prostitute. But this legislation too has had only limited success. Pheterson lists the range of third parties who can be caught up in 'antipimping laws': (1) managers hired by sex workers to oversee appointments; (2) boyfriend, girlfriends or husbands with whom sex workers share income and accommodation; (3) hotel managers who rent rooms to sex workers; (4) parents of sex workers who receive money from them; (5) men who force women to do sex work for money; and (6) men who entice women with promises of marriage or non-sex work and then coerce them into the sex industry. She adds:

> The last two examples are clear cases of abuse. However, antipimping laws mingle abusive acts with commercial acts with private choices. Most prostitutes are dependent upon

commercial agreements with third parties and many prostitutes have families who rely upon their income.

(1993: 45)

While the manifest function of such law may be to punish exploiting third parties, most notably brutal pimps, the latent function is to further harass women sex workers and their – frequently benign – associates.

Laws at once reflect, legitimate and reproduce social norms; and women sex workers can be said to infringe a number of deep-seated social norms associated with honour/dishonour. Pheterson (1993: 46) cites the following sources of *social dishonour*: (1) having sex with strangers; (2) having sex with multiple partners; (3) taking sexual initiativc and control and possessing expertise; (4) asking for money for sex; (5) being committed to satisfying impersonal male lust and fantasies; (6) being out alone on the streets at night dressed to attract male desire; and (7) being in the company of supposedly drunk or abusive men whom they either can handle ('common' or 'vulgar' women) or cannot handle ('victimized' women).

For many women sex workers 'being a prostitute' is not in itself shameful. They do not accept, even if they are not impervious to, society's ubiquitous cultural norms around (hetero-)sexual relations. Often they have their own sub-cultural, or counter-cultural, notions of honour/dishonour. These may be related to distinctions between 'good whores' and 'bad whores'. Good whores are variously defined as women who maintain a code of fair work, ask for money in advance, leave their clients feeling satisfied, use healthy practices like washing clients and insisting on condoms, remain emotionally (and sexually) detached, never provide services not negotiated beforehand, keep off alcohol and other drugs when working, and warn other women about dangerous or unreliable clients. Thus dishonour for many sex workers is not associated with sex work *per se*, but with a lack of competence and integrity in the conduct of work.

Social norms in relation to clients are much more ambiguous than are those in relation to sex workers. 'Whereas a whore is deemed dishonourable *as a woman*, the very criteria of unworthiness for the trick are also criteria of *manliness*' – for example, seeing a woman as a sex object, pursuing self-satisfaction without regard for her feelings, and paying for her body as for any (other) commodity (Pheterson 1993: 47). Often it is as if clients are culpable in public perception primarily, or only, for getting caught or being found out. Certainly, unlike sex workers, their identities are rarely 'spoiled' on exposure (Goffman 1968). Sex worker criticisms of clients tend to hinge on their hypocrisy: too often clients do business with sex workers in private and censure them in public.

The public stereotype of the pimp, the 'prototypical villain', is far more negative: 'a pimp is presumed to *exploit* women, in particular *white teenage* women, to *deceive* them, *addict* them to drugs, *batter* them, *rape* them, and *abandon* them' (Pheterson 1993: 48). Women sex workers object to presumptions that *all* women have pimps, that *all* pimps are mean and violent, and that *all* women are invariably helpless. 'Many' do not have pimps. It is in fact not known what proportion of sex workers do, although various estimates have been made. For example, McLeod (1982) estimates that about 75 per cent of women sex workers in Birmingham had pimps, with 'heavy' pimps – that is, men prone to violence and intimidation – more prevalent among street workers. She adds that having pimps is not so much indicative of women's helplessness as of 'their position as women – exacerbated by their criminal status' (1982: 44).

Psychological dishonour is often articulated in terms of either psychological or psycho-social *profiles* of women sex workers. Classically, the former describe 'a woman with a childhood of deprivation and abuse who is sexually frigid, hostile toward men, and latently or openly lesbian' (Pheterson 1993: 51). The latter typically maintain that women become sex workers either for the income prostitution provides or out of coercion. Both understate the heterogeneity of sex workers, which may be partly because most studies have been of street workers or of those in prison, where teenage and drug-using sex workers are over-represented. Rates of parental neglect and abuse are higher among teenage sex workers than among teenage non-sex workers. This difference is found too in adulthood, but it is less striking. As Pheterson (1993: 54) adds however: 'This is by no means to say that child sex abuse is not uncommon also among nonwhores or that there are not many whores who were not abused.' There is no evidence to support the view that sex workers are prone to frigidity; nor that they are more likely than non-sex workers to be lesbians or to be hostile to men.

The separation of love and sex which is considered deviant, or at least neurotic, in sex workers is recognized as normal in male clients. And since clients are not regarded as a deviant group, stereotypical perceptions of them are much more diffuse than are those of sex workers. After all, as Boyle (1994: 41) attests:

> There is no such thing as a typical punter. That is one of the few issues prostitutes and police agree on. Another fairly safe but maybe distressing bet is that a male member of your family, circle of friends or work colleagues has paid a prostitute for sex. Statistics from surveys carried out over the past few years suggest that up to one in five men have paid for some kind of sexual service at some time in their lives.

In the British *National Survey of Sexual Attitudes and Lifestyles*, 6.8 per cent of men reported having paid for sex with a woman at some time, and 1.8 per cent had done so within the last five years; but the authors argue that stigmatization might well have led to under-reporting (Wellings *et al.* 1994: 121).

Public perceptions of pimps are more graphic. Pheterson (1993: 56) points out that the profile of the pimp as 'a revengeful, impotent, violent latent homosexual man' may describe some pimps 'just as it describes some husbands'. Certainly many pimps are abusive. However recent research has revealed rather more male abuse in marriages than expected, and rather less male abuse in the sex industry *by pimps* than expected. Reports from women sex workers suggest that more abuse may be suffered from police officers and clients, especially on the streets, than from pimps. The English Collective of Prostitutes estimates that more than half sex workers have been raped by clients, although only one in twelve reports the attacks (Boyle 1994: 58). Sex workers are often protective of their pimps.

Ideological dishonour arises in relation to feminist critiques of prostitution. For many – but not all – feminists, prostitution represents:

> the ultimate objectification of women and the ultimate alienation of labour. Whores are thereby considered the prototype victims of patriarchy and capitalism. Empowerment within prostitution is, according to this analysis, an ideological contradiction in terms . . . Women who claim self-determination *as prostitutes* lose victim status and ideological sympathy.
>
> (Pheterson 1993: 57–8)

Not surprisingly the tensions between sex workers and feminists can be marked, with the 'subtlety' of the feminist slogan '*Against* prostitution. *For* prostitutes' lost on the former (Scambler *et al.* 1990: 269; see also Bell 1985).

If this commentary on Pheterson's dissection of the whore stigma has corrected some stereotypical misperceptions of women sex workers, then it has served its purpose. Some of what McCall and Simmons refer to as errors of commission, omission and of the attribution of fixed characteristics have been exposed; and, perhaps most significantly, the nature of the association between stereotypical error and the projects of key stereotypers in societies like Britain, namely, *male* norm- and law-makers and enforcers, has been registered.

THE MUNDANE NATURE OF SEX WORK

Reference might be made at this juncture to what might be termed the *paradox of attention*. This asserts that much of the notoriety and excitement generated around prostitution is a function less of what sex workers do than of the attention paid to it. It is evident, for example, that many of the objections to sex work, feminist and non-feminist alike, apply equally well to other forms of work to which far less attention and indignation is directed. In fact, women sex workers and the lives they lead are far more mundane than is implied in the excesses of attention and stereotype. They are for the most part *ordinary* women systematically and ideologically misrepresented – in line with the projects of those who do so – as extraordinary. It is to the mundanity of sex workers' lives that we now turn. For convenience, the necessarily attenuated discussion is subsumed under the following headings: *recruitment*, *patterns of work*, *lifestyle* and *projects*.

There are many factors predisposing to *recruitment* to the sex industry, but relative poverty has generally been regarded as the most salient. McLeod (1982: 26) argues persuasively that 'women's entry into prostitution is characterized by an act of resistance to the experience of relative poverty or the threat of it'. In an Australian survey as many as 97 per cent of women questioned gave money as their reason for becoming sex workers, and 85 per cent of these spoke of 'economic survival' (Perkins and Bennett 1985). Several studies have suggested that a high proportion, perhaps 70 per cent, may support homes and children (in which case control over hours is another attraction). Certainly the income the industry can generate is a key motivation.

In introducing their study of sex workers in Oslo, Hoigard and Finstad (1992: 15) claim that it is 'established knowledge' in international research on prostitution that women sex workers are recruited 'from the working class and the lumenproletariat', adding that 'their backgrounds are also marked by irregular home lives and adjustment difficulties in school and in their working lives'. Their own 26 interviewees fitted this pattern, and no fewer than 23 of them had experience of institutional care or detention: 15 of the 23 had one or more stays in institutions before engaging in sex work. Hoigard and Finstad (1992: 16) cite in detail the case of 'Anita', who had been 'institutionalized 12 times' by the age of 20. They emphasize both that many of the young women they interviewed had already been rejected 'by normal society' *before* becoming sex workers, and that institutions can be important 'training grounds' for sex workers. 'In institutions many young people in trouble are stowed together like surplus wreckage. They often run away together, without money. What could be more natural than that they exchange knowledge about ways to survive?' (Hoigard and Finstad 1992: 16.)

The small Oslo sample may not be representative, but personal biography is certainly relevant to recruitment. While writers like Pheterson have properly sought to debunk male myths about the 'psychopathology of the prostitute', it remains the case that women sex workers are more likely than non-sex workers to have had poor relationships with their fathers, and, to a lesser extent, to have been abused by them; to have become emotionally distanced from their families of origin, and therefore from family influence and disapproval; and to have developed strong independent personalities. What needs to be stressed, however, is that insofar as personal biography does predispose to sex work, it does so 'only in connection with local conditions, such as the existence of a number of women working in prostitution and more structural forces such as employment opportunities' (McLeod 1982: 30). Peer contact can be an important feature of a 'drift' into sex work, bringing both opportunity and training.

There is a neglected group of women too, proportionately more of them off-street workers from middle-class backgrounds, who exercise conscious choice in turning to sex work. The appropriateness of referring to 'conscious choice' here might be disputed, but there can be no question that *even* women confronted with relative poverty, primed by their personal biographies and with peers in sex work can take conscious decisions to enter or not to enter the sex industry; and some women decide to engage in sex work outside the sway of all such predisposing circumstances. Indeed, the benefits as opposed to the costs of sex work for women are frequently understated. Of those in Perkins and Bennett's (1985) survey, 24 per cent said they liked the work, variously citing its financial rewards, the freedom and autonomy it affords, and the satisfaction of providing a service, all of which sentiments have been echoed in the bestselling autobiography of the American sex worker, Dolores French (1988). The same attitudes are reflected in comments made to the author by 'Gillian' and 'Sarah' respectively:

> It suits me down to the ground to do two hours work and get the same money that most people get for doing 40 hours . . . it's easy money. . . . I wouldn't go back to scrabbling around on £50 a week again.

> I choose when I work. I choose my clients. I say 'No' if I'm busy. . . . I don't feel as though I'm trapped in any sort of vicious circle of work, or being pressurized by any men at all. . . . Prostitution is giving yourself and your attention to someone for a period of time. . . . You're offering more than just a body: you're offering an experience which usually they remember quite well.

At the time of interview 'Sarah', who like 'Gillian' worked through a London escort agency, was in fact seeing one client per week to fund her way through a postgraduate degree in Fine Arts (Scambler *et al.* 1990: 23).

Patterns of work vary in the sex industry. In part this occurs by type and location of work: thus the routines of street workers, hotel or bar workers, workers in saunas or massage parlours, workers with escort agencies and workers in flats and brothels all differ considerably and with some degree of consistency. It is often dramatic and exceptional breaks with these routines, especially if they involve clients who are violent or display bizarre fetishes, that make journalistic headlines or sell books (McCrae 1992); but for many women in the sex industry work tends towards a rather dull, tense and sometimes inebriated monotony characterized by a great deal of waiting around (see Jaget 1980). As 'Connie' puts it, 'whoring is boring, but lucrative' (Taylor 1991: 17).

If sex workers are not unique in finding much of their work monotonous, no more are they in developing *instrumental* attitudes to both work and clients. Many just want to get their work task, the sexual (or other) act, over in minimum time ('A good customer is a fast customer'); many cut themselves off mentally for the duration of contact ('I try to think of something else. Plan what I am going to do with the money'); and many, too, forbid the intimacy of kissing and see the condom as a barrier, real and symbolic ('He will never be able to reach me, I think to myself. It is like the condom guarantees that he will never touch me') (Jarvinen 1993: 144).

Stereotyping remains hazardous however. Caring relationships with 'regulars' are not unknown, and women occasionally have orgasms with clients (French 1988). Jarvinen (1993: 143), who found that as many as half the sex workers interviewed 'had been sexually interested in some of their customers', cites the following account:

> Fond of, well . . . it can be a type of person that makes me feel a certain way . . . like that man I told you about. He came to me a few times and something happened between us. . . . We have a stronger relationship . . . a sexual relationship. . . . It is not only for the money. . . . We make love fully and completely, holding nothing back.

But such accounts tend to be rare and are normally regarded within the industry as 'unprofessional'.

The requests for sexual (and other) acts made by clients reveal a staggering variety of tastes and needs. The more exotic, 'kinky', dangerous or – to use Perkins and Bennett's term – 'gut-turning' seem to have been laid endlessly before us and will not be detailed here. Faced with such requests, the attitudes of some women remain instrumental: 'If a person is crazy enough to want to pay me to piss on him, then he is welcome to do so'; 'If he wants to be whipped, the disgusting old coot, then I might as well be the one holding the whip' (Jarvinen 1993: 145). But for others, their own *code of practice*, which typically extends well beyond an insistence on hygiene and condom-use, proscribes sexual (and other) acts outside a pre-defined set of categories. Thus 'Gillian', quoted earlier, explained that she would not permit clients to revert to babyhood and don nappies because she judged them to be in need of therapy not reinforcement. Many women in fact will not sanction acts which they see as deeply degrading. As 'Helen' told Silver (1993: 87):

> As a prostitute you've got to be comfortable with what you take on, otherwise it becomes too stressful. If you keep on pushing yourself into situations which you dread or find repulsive then you do suffer psychological damage.

In the early 1980s McLeod (1982: 69–72) estimated that about half to three-quarters of sex workers' clients wanted 'straightforward sexual intercourse, whatever else they wanted'; about a fifth sought the passive experience of 'domination', a finding even more marked in earlier American studies by Winick (1962) and Stein (1974); and about a quarter wanted to dress up as a woman. It may be that after a decade of public awareness of AIDS as a heterosexual threat, the proportion of women willing to provide, or clients intent on procuring, sexual intercourse has declined, although decisive data are unavailable. Certainly some women have redefined the categories of service they are prepared to offer, some entirely eliminating 'genital sex work' (Morgan 1988).

Like patterns of work, the graded *fees* women charge for sexual services vary. At what many commentators and women themselves define as the lower end of the market, for example on the streets or 'working the windows', 'Samantha's' rates are probably typical:

> £10 for hand relief, £15–20 for straight sex, £20 for oral, £25 for oral and sex or strip and sex, £30 for strip, oral and sex, and those wanting to spend 30 minutes of their time with her will have to fork out £40.
>
> (Boyle 1994: 145)

These rates may be contrasted with those charged by women at the upper end of the market, for example with exclusive escort agencies or madames or independently. Boyle contends that it is women who work independently, inconspicuous and grossly under-represented in research studies, who tend to enjoy the highest incomes. One of Boyle's (1994: 12–18) interviewees, 'Diana', is 30 years old and occupies a mews cottage close to Regents Park in London. She estimates that 95 per cent of her work is 'specialized': a dominatrix, her work revolves around fantasy and S&M (sado-masochism). For clients unsure what they want she offers a 'taste of everything' during a 90-minute session for £500. Despite massive overheads (rent, equipment, maid, 'card boys', etc.), she makes up to £1,500 profit a week.

Another commonsense assumption is that women sex workers' *lifestyles* are determined or decisively marked by their livelihoods. While this may be emphatically true for some women, it is doubtless true for no higher proportion of sex workers than for other workers. And nor should circumstances and behaviours sometimes associated with the sex industry, such as drug habits, be confounded with sex work itself. Again, the paradox of attention 'misses' the ordinary and the commonplace.

In fact, unexceptionally, most women sex workers spend much of their time preoccupied with the day-to-day business of living and supporting and maintaining households. This aspect of their biographies and *projects* for the future remains largely uninvestigated and unreported.

Ward, Day and colleagues (1993) took some pains to recruit women from all sectors of the sex industry in London for their study of health issues. They are careful not to claim representativeness for their sample of 280 women, but aspects of the profile of sex workers it affords are interesting, not least because two-thirds of them worked in off-street locations. Of the sample, 39 per cent had experience of schooling beyond the statutory leaving age of 16; 8 per cent of the women were current or past injecting drug users; rather more, 19 per cent, reported the use of injected drugs *either* by themselves *or* by their sexual partners.

As far as drug use is concerned, this profile might usefully be compared with that found in the profusion of studies of the sex industry focusing exclusively on street workers. Consider, for example, a study in Glasgow by Green and his colleagues (1993). Of the 63 women in their sample, no fewer than 81 per cent were injecting drug users, the most commonly used drugs being heroin and temazepam. Predictably, most studies report higher rates of injecting drug use on the streets than in off-street locations (Scambler and Scambler 1995); and it is of course conspicuous street workers who are the most frequent objects of interest and investigation.

Stereotypically, the principal project of the sex worker, namely, the rapid accumulation of money to support a subsequent decent and respectable lifestyle outside the sex industry, is doomed to fail: women, it is said, neither save nor emerge psychologically unscathed from the sex industry. This stereotype receives some reinforcement from research on the experiences of ageing, drug-using or otherwise 'trapped' sex workers. But how much research has been done with women – be they full-time, part-time or occasional casual workers – who have made good money from the industry *and departed from it unscathed* to return *incognito* to the community? A search has revealed none.

SOME THESES ABOUT SEX WORKERS

The object of this chapter has been to identify and comment on errors embodied in pivotal myths and stereotypes surrounding the sex industry and sex workers. Key themes have been the understandable but misleading propensity to extrapolate from often impressionistic or anecdotal observations about small numbers of conspicuous street workers to *all* sex workers; and, more broadly, the paradox of attention. In this final section five specific qualifications to common misconceptions of women in the sex industry are offered by way of summary.

The first point to reiterate is that women sex workers are a heterogeneous body of workers, most of whom diverge markedly from the popular stereotype of the sex worker as a street worker who is vulgar, without morality, and situated in a milieu characterized by drug use, violence, anomie and hopelessness. As one university-educated escort worker stressed to the author, most women sex workers are invisible off-street workers, many of them autonomous and successful enough to evade public and (even) self-labelling as outsiders or outcasts.

Second, it is inappropriate to characterize sex workers as passive 'victims' of psycho-pathological or socio-pathological circumstance. To do so is to provide yet another instance of the 'gender-prescribed passivity' over which many feminists have taken umbrage (see Naffine 1987). Adler (1975: 83) may be overstating her case, but her insistence that sex workers are no longer passive objects of male needs is apt: 'like other modern women, today's prostitute is better educated, better accepted, and more independent of men'. Certainly the respectful premise that women are active, autonomous agents is no less justified in relation to sex workers than in relation to other female workers. There is evidence, too, that women sex workers, unlike many rent-boys, exercise considerable control over their encounters with clients (Perkins and Bennett 1985).

Third, it is erroneous to judge sex workers to be lacking in moral sensibilities or commitment. The author was told by one off-street worker: 'We have our ethical code, just like doctors; it's no different.' In fact, most sex workers have what amounts to a code of practice, governing everything from condom-use to the delineation of services for hire. Nor, it can be assumed, are sex workers any more predisposed to flout social norms or laws than other people, that is, with the exception of those which embody the 'double-standard' of patriarchy to limit their own capacity to provide professional – as opposed to amateur – sexual services.

A fourth qualification to the familiar characterization of sex workers concerns their reflexivity. Rather than being conditioned dupes, sex workers require resourcefulness and expertise to cope day to day and to sustain their livelihoods. In acquiring these attributes there is little they do not learn also of the hypocrisy, fallibility and 'deviance' of 'respectable' men and, circuitously, of the institutions in which they serve. One brothel-owner listed to the author numerous peers, MPs, judges and men of business and the City among her clientele; and an escort worker similarly detailed the regular visits of one member of each House at Westminster and of their purchases. Neither was censorious, but each was able to articulate an attenuated but clear and compelling account of the continuing exercise of male influence in essentially patriarchal social institutions.

Finally, there needs to be recognition of an innovative or pioneering dimension to women sex workers' norm-breaking. This idea might be developed in relation to a recent thesis of Giddens (1992). He argues that the potential exists in 'high modernity' for a sustained challenge to patriarchal structures and cultures, a potential nourished by such factors as a female life expectancy well beyond the year, of child-rearing; the deskilling of housework; access to education and the higher echelons of the labour market; the availability of contraception and divorce; and – most relevant here – what he terms *plastic sexuality*, that is, sexuality freed from its intrinsic relation to reproduction. The creation of plastic sexuality, he contends, was a precondition of the sexual revolution of recent decades. This revolution has two main components: first, there have been new gains, built on a century of struggle, in female sexual autonomy; and second, there has been a flourishing of homosexuality, male and female. The sexual revolution, in short, constitutes a challenge to what Brittan (1989) calls 'hierarchic heterosexuality'.

Not only have women sex workers figured in the 'century of

struggle', but some might be said to be contributing to sexual emancipation by integrating plastic sexuality with the reflexive project of self. Thus the prostitute activist Helen Buckingham told Silver (1993: 78):

> I challenged the current supposition that men could have women when they felt like it, with no obligation, and that women enjoyed the sex, enjoyed giving themselves, enjoyed being walked over, enjoyed being used, enjoyed being disposed of. They thought that this is all part of the feminine personality: women are masochistic by nature and they like this. And to meet a woman who said, 'No, I'm not like that and I don't like it, but this is a bloody good way to earn a living' was terribly, terribly threatening.

It is autonomy and reciprocity that are crucial here. There are women who *choose* the rewards than can attend sex work, such as higher pay than most women and many men in more orthodox employment, foreign travel and unusual freedom; and some of these women enjoy their work. And if much female sex work yet remains deeply symptomatic of patriarchy, this does not prevent many women from dominating most of their encounters with most of their clients. There is assertion and resistance to patriarchy even here.

The contention here that any consideration of the sex industry and sex workers should start with the *presumption* that women are individualistic, active and wilful, moral, reflexive and insightful, as well as potential innovators with respect to patriarchal norms, should *not* of course be read as a denial that *any* of their number conform to the popular stereotype of the sex worker. As anybody who has researched or worked with women sex workers is only too painfully aware, the sex industry can exact a terrible price, including life itself. The extent to which the unacceptable price some sex workers pay is a function of the stigma, marginality and harassment which is their routine, but contingent, lot is a theme tackled more directly in other contributions to this volume.

Chapter 6

Boyfriends, 'pimps' and clients

Jean Faugier and Mary Sargeant

INTRODUCTION

This chapter describes the characteristics of clients and pimps and embeds these traits within the social, historical and cultural dimensions of prostitution. It examines the stereotypes of female prostitutes as victims of coercive male pimps and the impact of crack-cocaine on 1990s street prostitution. It highlights the relationships between prostitutes and their sexual partners and addresses the impact of social marginalization and the law and the need for risk reduction strategies. Faugier's (1996) study of 50 drug-using and 100 non-drug-using prostitutes working in the Manchester area will be used as a current example within this context. The study included interviews with 120 male clients and focused particularly on the sexual and drug-related risk behaviour of the women and their clients, attempting to provide some understanding of their lives, decisions and needs in terms of health care.

CULTURAL STEREOTYPES OF FEMALE PROSTITUTES AS VICTIMS OF COERCIVE MALE PIMPS

Boyle (1994) claims that, if prostitution is the world's oldest profession, then pimping must be the runner-up. It is currently estimated that between 80 per cent and 95 per cent of all prostitution is pimp controlled (Barry 1995). Giobbe (1987), in her study of prostitution in Minneapolis, USA, reported that 53 per cent of the women she interviewed were brought to it by a pimp and 90 per cent had pimps whilst in prostitution. The link between the pimp and the prostitute is depicted as the most inexplicable and repulsive element of commercialized sex, a relationship based on unilateral exploitation, polygamy and criminality. Although these rela-tionships vary in terms of commerciality, duration, selectivity, promiscuity and emotionality (Jarvinen 1993: 34), violence has traditionally been viewed as the means by which pimps have controlled and exploited women, along with such guises as pretending that they care about the women, playing on their vulnerability by comparing them to other women who work for them and getting them on drugs (Boyle 1994). Beatings, rape and even murder of prostitutes by pimps is not uncommon and the Council for Prostitution Alternatives, in Portland, Oregon, reported that of 179 women in their programme who left prostitution in 1990–91, almost half were raped by pimps an average of sixteen times per year. They also calculated that, out of 55 women in their programme, 63 per cent were horribly beaten by pimps an average of 58 times a year. At worst, pimping has been defined as a condition of female sexual slavery:

> A lover, husband, or boyfriend who promotes the sexual exploitation and commodification of women is a pimp, and together, pimping and procuring are amongst the most ruthless practices of male power and sexual dominance. These practices go far beyond the merchandising of women's bodies for the market that demands them; they crystallize misogyny in acts of male hatred of femaleness as rendered into a commodity for whom the marketer and the purchaser have contempt.
>
> (Barry 1995: 199)

Pimps, regardless of their race, or their ways of operating, have pimping rules for control over women in prostitution (Barry 1995). In his autobiography, the notorious pimp Iceberg Slim gives his first rule of thumb in pimping:

> The best pimps keep a steel lid on their emotions and I was one of the iciest . . . any good pimp is his own best company. His inner life is so rich with cunning and scheming to out-think his whores.
>
> (Slim 1969)

In 1989, the Goteborg Prostitution group in Sweden described a pimp procuring scenario which created the conditions by which a woman ended up prostituting herself. The pimp began using the facade of friendship and romance. He then started familiarizing the woman with the subject of hustling and started seductive coaxing until she finally decided to go onto the streets. Similarly, in their field research on pimps, Christina and Richard Milner (1972) examined the process of 'seasoning' and they found that pimps wanted loyalty and obedience from a women, more than her body, and for that they needed to change her identity:

> You create a different environment. It's a brainwashing process; the whole thing is creativity. When you turn a chick out, you take away every set of values and morality she had previously and create a different environment.
>
> (Steve, pimp)

To test the popular notions of talk, drugs and violence tactics used by pimps to force women to work as prostitutes, Armstrong (1983) designed a study using participant observation within a Port Authority bus terminal, a likely recruitment site, and a survey of Port Authority police officers, to gain opinions of experts. However, his research findings were contradictory and he concludes that pimps play only a minor role in the recruitment process. The cultural stereotype of prostitutes as victims of coercive male pimps is complicated by the fact that liaisons are seldom one-dimensional from the perspectives of the involved parties. From the prostitute's point of view the traditional depiction of the pimp may be oversimplified and poorly reflects her reality. She may perceive a unique and interdependent alliance, where her pimp is an integral part of her social network and often her security system (Jarvinen 1993: 34).

Faugier (1994: 56) nevertheless argues that it is dangerous to misconstrue these women as self-assured, when in fact they are often vulnerable, damaged both physically and psychologically, and may well be lacking necessary sexual skills. In their investigation of abuse of female prostitutes in San Francisco, Silbert and Pines (1982) document a cycle of victimization which starts with physical, emotional and sexual abuse at home and continues with extensive physical and sexual abuse, on and off the job, after entering prostitution. Out of the 200 juvenile and adult current and former prostitutes interviewed, 70 per cent reported that sexual exploitation affected their decision to become a prostitute and 96 per cent started prostitution after running away from home as a result of these abuses. Once on the streets, 70 per cent were victimized both by customers and pimps; they were beaten, robbed, raped and abused. Similar findings are reported by Hardesty and Greif (1994), based on two years of therapeutic work with female drug users who were also HIV positive and in methadone maintenance programmes. The authors present accounts of some of the women's experiences relating to sexual and physical abuse and neglect at the hands of family members, friends and strangers, often as a continuation of a cycle of abuse from childhood. This had left an indelible impression of worthlessness which the women went on to carry into their current relationships with parents, friends, lovers and children. These women were also frequently involved with men who took advantage of them; similarly, those who worked as prostitutes were often beaten up or robbed.

PIMPS AND DEALERS – THE DRUG AS PIMP

Crack-cocaine has had an enormous impact on the context of street prostitutes' relationships with men and has intensified the link between drugs and the female–male power relationships on the streets (Miller 1995). A study undertaken by Goldstein *et al.* (1992) implies that the arrival of illegal drugs, and in particular crack-cocaine, onto the streets of Chicago has directly and indirectly affected the drugs/prostitution nexus by lowering the price for street prostitutes, altering the social status of cocaine, and increasing the level of social disorganization in illicit street activities. The authors argue that the current illicit distribution of crack-cocaine and its presence on the street prostitution scene is comparable with the liquor industry in Chicago in the early twentieth century, when prostitutes were employed to attract customers. The role played in prostitution by traditional pimps and madams (who were often vigorously opposed to the use of drugs by working girls) has now declined and is being replaced by drug dealers representing new economic interests. Thus Goldstein *et al.* (1992) note that the sleazy illegal saloons of Chicago are now being upstaged by the contemporary crack or smoke house.

The incarcerated prostitutes in Miller's (1995) study in Columbus, Ohio, all claimed to be independent of any one man acting as a pimp and argued that they had eliminated their reliance on pimps. Indeed, the prostitutes to whom Miller spoke uniformly believed that drugs had replaced pimps in most women's lives: 'It was commonly believed that crack-cocaine had altered traditional pimp–prostitute relationships, lessening the role of the pimp on the streets as a result of the prostitutes' overriding concern with chasing crack.' Similar findings have been reported by Inciardi *et al.* (1993) and Ratner (1993).

Although it may be true that drug addicted women may be less appealing in terms of profit for pimps, Miller (1995) argues that the assertion that prostitutes are now independent of men on the streets remains largely untrue: 'Although they were free from the exploitation of what they perceived as traditional pimping relations, they remained in a highly exploitable position on the streets as women involved in the largely male dominated drug scene.' In fact, drug dealers acted in exactly the same fashion as pimps had previously, in that nearly all the women working the streets handed the vast majority of their earnings to them and still had to have sex with them. McKeganey and Barnard (1992b: 76) in their study of female prostitutes in Glasgow, report that whilst they found no evidence to suggest that the women were working for male pimps, many of the women had males in attendance to protect them who were themselves drug users and with whom they had sexual relationships.

According to Rosenbaum (1981), women are likely to become initiated into illegal drugs by means of a male relationship; this was also shown by Klee *et al.* (1990). Stephens (1991) argues that, once initiated, women continue to buy their supply often from the man who got them into drugs, and that they also tend to develop larger, more dependent habits more quickly than most men. Drug use among women is consistently perceived as more deviant than among men, due to the latter's higher rate of use. Indeed, as Inciardi *et al.* (1993) found, the higher up the hierarchy you go, the more the gender balance tilts in favour of men. Ratner (1993) and Fagan (1994) also claim that women are much more likely to be found on the lower social ladders of the drugs world, partly because they are seen as uncontrolled drug users who are willing to trade sex for drugs, but also and more importantly because of their access to supplies. As a consequence of their domestic situations, female users are unlikely to have access to the lucrative world of drug dealing which is reserved as an almost exclusively male activity. Williams (1992) and French (1993) also highlight the low status of women users in the social networks of the street drugs scene; they both point out the presence of abstinent male dealers on the very highest rungs of that scene. Fagan further notes: that their absence from the ranks of dealers relegates women to a lower status and their reliance on sex – a commodity under their control – as a means of barter for money or drugs is equated with a loss of sexual control.

These gender relations are both sealed and maintained by the active part played by violence at street level within an illegal drugs world controlled by a male-dominated hierarchy (Inciardi *et al.* 1993), where drug dealers' reputations are often built on violence and the willingness to use firearms. This violence is understood in terms of the respect it earns, and the low status and weaker physical power of women means they can expect no respect from male users or dealers (Bourgois and Dunlap 1993). Thus, the drug dealer–prostitute relationship could in fact be perceived as less beneficial to women than pimping due to their structural dependence on the male dealers for their supply of drugs. Whereas Boyle (1994) found that traditional pimps, whilst treating women in a violent and abusive way, were inclined to limit such abuse if it started to interfere with the woman's ability to earn the money, the association with drugs now means that, no matter what state the woman might be in, she will still go out on the streets because she needs the money for drugs:

> The rock is the pimp. . . . We go there, we do all this, we get all this money, first person we run to is the dope man. The rock is the pimp. . . . So that's why they call us strawberries, 'cause we get the rocks and we will have oral sex, have you, have your brother too, all at the same time to get this cocaine.
>
> (Interview with crack-using prostitute, in Feucht 1993: 97)

The development of the drug as pimp has provided men with a new means of status attainment through the sexual degradation of women (Bourgois and Dunlap 1993; Feldman *et al.* 1993; Ouellet *et al.* 1993). The hierarchies which have previously structured the world of prostitution from high-class call girls down to street workers have given way to prostitution with no limits:

> the young girls who usually get drugs from a pimp and are then sent on the street, they do everything. They cannot care less. They are so broken in spirit and body, they don't have the strength to take care of themselves. . . . Today they are rather isolated, they completely surrender to their pimp.
>
> (Interview with older German prostitute, from Schwarzer, cited in Barry 1995: 40)

Miller (1995) describes how the female drug-using prostitutes in her study constantly received abuse from the men involved in the drug scene, which frequently resulted in the women being badly beaten. During the course of Faugier's (1996) study, a number of women suffered extremely violent attacks by male clients and boyfriends and were on a number of occasions robbed of their earnings. One woman was beaten with a cricket bat by her drug-using boyfriend because she refused to go out to work the streets at 9 a.m. in order to supply his habit; another was so badly attacked by a client with a knife that she needed to be admitted to intensive care and, for a while, it was thought she would lose her arm. Most disturbingly, one contact was murdered during the period of data collection. She was severely mutilated and found in plastic bags in a local lake; no one has ever been charged with her murder. However, even though other women were shocked and distressed by this murder, they continued to work.

In an attempt to differentiate between the men who control female prostitutes, Miller (1995) distinguishes between a 'man' and a pimp, according to the number of prostitutes they have. She then extends this to a continuum in which one extreme constitutes the pimp who manages a group of women in a relatively bureaucratic way, while the other signifies the husband or lover of the women. Barry (1995) agrees that there is a continuum between a pimp and 'a man', but highlights that the real question is the extent to which he is involved in a relationship with the prostitute and whether she is subjected to sexual exploitation *from him* and/or *because of him*. Male-dominated ideologies surrounding the image of women as 'Madonna' or 'whore' are ingrained within our society. This double standard approach to sexuality and the prejudices which permeate society have long permitted the victimization of women by the power and cruelty of men. There is a fine line between men who are traditionally perceived as using women as sexual commodities for money and men who pay money to use women as sexual commodities:

> It is a fact of prostitution that once a woman 'tricks' for a man, she is never again not his 'whore'. He thinks of her as such, whether or not he is otherwise known to her as husband, lover, brother or father.
>
> (Barry 1995: 198)

RELATIONSHIPS BETWEEN PROSTITUTES AND THEIR SEXUAL PARTNERS, PRIVATE PARTNERS AND CLIENTS, REGULAR AND CASUAL

In contrast to traditional prostitute/pimp relationships and non-commercial relationships, where the power balance is generally weighted towards the male partner (Holland *et al.* 1990), the prostitute/client relationship is one where the female attempts to establish control. In selling their services, they would try to determine the sexual services on offer, the price and the place of the sexual act. However, underlying effects of violence and intimidation as well as the influence of drugs may make the issue of control potentially problematic (McKeganey and Barnard 1992a: 84).

One way that prostitutes attempt to take control is through the use of condoms. Prostitutes feel at risk from AIDS from clients and they have been found to use condoms more frequently with clients than with steady partners (Dorfman *et al.* 1992). Prostitutes describe sexual contacts with clients in unemotional, business-like terms where condoms are valued both for symbolic and purely practical reasons (McKeganey and Barnard 1990: 86). Through her work with prostitutes in Vienna, Girtler (1984) also found that prostitutes tried to distance themselves personally and internally from their clients to counteract the degradation of being merchandise. Personal pleasure was not sought but rather denied since they typically separated their private from their client customers. Similarly, in their cohort study of female prostitutes attending a genito-urinary clinic in London, Day and Ward (1990) noted how condoms acted as important ideological tools for creating and maintaining boundaries between private and public sexual encounters. This attitude is well exemplified by a prostitute interviewed in their study:

> It's all right for you [Sophie Day]. You don't work with a gross of condoms by the bed, six days a week. How could I use condoms outside work? . . . the mere thought of putting a condom on a boyfriend or watching him put it on just leaves me cold. I'd rather not have sex.

However, the formation of this very real distinction in terms of behaviour between clients and husbands or boyfriends itself creates a high-risk element for both parties, considering that the non-working lives of prostitutes, which are not associated with high rates of partner exchange or directly with the sale of sex, commonly involve unprotected sex (Day and Ward 1988). Faugier (1996) found that even with those prostitutes who strived to use condoms in their working encounters, condom use with regular sexual partners was very low and this was perceived by a number of non-drug users, particularly sauna workers, as a positive means of distinguishing between work and personal sexual experiences. The extent of the problem was evident in Day and Ward's (1990) study, where many of the women attending the clinic with infections immediately attributed them to their private partners. Even more worryingly, half the women from the study who had boyfriends reported that they knew that these men had other sexual partners, with whom, it was suspected, condoms were not used. In addition, Faugier (1996) found that drug-using women were even less likely than non-drug-using women to use condoms with other casual sexual partners due to pressure from partners and feelings of powerlessness. Barry (1995) concurs that any ability of women to distance and dissociate themselves to sustain some aspect of themselves has collapsed in street prostitution of the 1990s with the introduction of crack (cocaine).

However, studies suggest that the distinction between public and private sex may sometimes become blurred by superficial judgements on issues such as cleanliness, reliability and kindness (Faugier 1994: 58). In his study of male clients in Camden, New Jersey, Leonard (1990) found that clients often want to develop a relationship of trust and intimacy with a prostitute, in which the need for the use of condoms is lessened by a false sense that the woman is somehow special. Many prostitutes are less likely to insist upon condom use as they get to know clients better, or they become 'regulars', paying to see the same woman repeatedly. In between the casual or new client and the private partner, the 'regular client' assures women of an income, and may allow them to establish themselves as self-employed business women rather than employees (Walkowitz 1980: 197). Payment becomes evaluated differently than with casual clients and may take the form of material help, protection, transport, or rent. 'Regulars' may also be involved in the women's personal lives and occasionally turn into private partners (Day and Ward 1990: 71).

DIFFERENT TYPES OF CLIENTS AND CLIENT NEEDS AND DEMANDS

In her study, Faugier (1996) found that the clients contacted represented a mainly British, white, married and employed group of men with an average age of 39. Many were employed in professional or managerial positions and self-employed. A large number came from a much higher social class than the women and were currently in a much more advantaged position socially and economically:

> A lot of them are married. They come for things the wife won't do, or they come rather than have an affair: no commitment, you see. . . . This is not going to lead to me expecting a wedding ring, is it? . . . I find they are mostly business types, especially the ones who want domination stuff . . . I find they are the ones in the boss position. They dish it out all day, see, I think they like a bit back. . . . It turns them on, a woman shouting at them.
>
> (Maria, aged 28, drug user)

> It's basically the young guy that is either on his way to a club or on his way home from a club. He can't be bothered with the chatting up. He doesn't want to pick a girl up, then all evening pay for her drinks on the off chance that she may or she may not; and if she does, the next time he's in that pub, she is giving him a load of hassle like: 'Why didn't you phone?' and all that. Or it's the married man whose wife is pregnant or in the menopause or something, the middle-aged guy who is not sure he can still do it, you know.
>
> (Karine, aged 33, drug user)

> You get the lads that will bring their mate down from his stag night and pay for him, you know. You get the really old man who will walk round for an hour talking to all the girls and then he will pick one. They are just basically lonely, and he will pick the one who was the friendliest to him; she might have a face like the back of a bus, it won't matter, that will be the one he will go for.
>
> (Cathy, aged 21, drug user)

The majority of men reported approaching prostitutes on the streets, and many expressed the need to experience risk, to themselves, as an important element of using prostitutes:

> I've met some really nice people, through to top businessmen and others who are really pure arse-holes. They come in here and they think they can treat you like shit. You get loads of hassle not to use condoms, and I say: 'You're not coming in here doing that, so you can tell your mates on the building-site tomorrow.' You get it from all sides, though, really: the businessmen, the married men and the lower end of the market.
>
> (Michelle, non-drug user, aged 19 (sauna))

Faugier (1996) found that despite the fact that a significant number of men were buying anal and unprotected vaginal and oral sex from female prostitutes, only a minority ever visited genito-urinary clinics or had an HIV test. A number also said that they were unable to enjoy or, in some cases, actually perform sex with a condom. These accounts are supported by male clients in Leonard's (1990) study:

> Why should I use a rubber for a blowjob? Even if a woman has sores in her mouth, how's that gonna get in me unless I have a cut?
>
> If a woman uses a rubber I won't date her again.

Although there is very little work available on this topic, similar findings concerning this lack of ability to address issues of risk have been reported. From their pilot study of 30 male clients, Chetwynd and Plumridge (1994) found that the men took a passive role in terms of protection from infection, rarely if ever providing the condom, and were often involved in other casual relationships outside prostitution in which condom use was even less likely. McKeganey and Barnard (1992a) also uncovered a wide range of risk behaviour which clients were involved in alongside a limited acknowledgement on their part of any need for health care or caution.

This lack of ability to address issues of risk seems evident in other work which has examined attitudes of men who attend genito-urinary clinics. Sherr and Hedge (1990) surveyed 260 attenders at a sexually transmitted disease clinic to examine sexual behaviour, condom use and appraisal of risk, and to determine whether situational factors in the last sexual encounters were predictive of condom use. Risk exposure among respondents was consistently high despite messages about safe sex and risk of infection and there was consistent evidence of unprotected anal and vaginal intercourse. Difficulties with condoms were widespread and fell into both physical and psychological categories. Accounts from prostitutes have confirmed that clients often request sex without a condom for which they were prepared to pay extra money or deliberately try to burst or remove condoms:

> You get asked every night for it without a condom, some guys'll offer £200 without one in a hotel . . . no, no, they're no'usual but I mean there's not one type of guy. I mean they could be really rich or just regular kinds of guy, like just out the dancin' and wantin' a bit of business, but when you go to get the condom they're goin' 'Oh no, turn it up, I'm no wearing one of them.'
>
> (prostitute in the Glasgow red-light district, McKeganey *et al.* 1990: 78)

The same study reported that drug-using women were likely to be less discerning when it came to resisting the inducement of extra financial reward accompanying the requests for unprotected sex. This relates back to the issue of the drug as pimp and the urgency of the prostitutes to earn money to fuel their drug habits. However, as against their unwillingness to use condoms, Leonard (1990) found male clients were more cautious in terms of risk protection in their attempt to avoid drug dependent sex workers and only approach those they perceived as 'clean'. Many of the respondents believed that they could avoid infection by carefully selecting a prostitute who looked 'healthy' and admitted to selecting sex partners, inexperienced or occasional prostitutes and those who did not appear to be on drugs:

> Decent, clean. I look to see if there are sores over her mouth, brown spots, fever blisters. . . . These mean she has AIDS.
>
> (I) try and reduce the risk by choosing the right girl . . . try to choose women who don't look like they are prostitutes.
>
> No dope fiends. If she's on drugs, I won't do anything.

A similar risk protection strategy was also used by the prostitutes themselves. McKeganey and Barnard (1992a) found that some of the non-IDU women in their study would refuse to provide sexual services to a client whom they knew or suspected of having contacted an IDU prostitute. They found that there was considerable friction between the non-IDU and IDU women, which stemmed from accusations that the drug users accepted unprotected sex for more money and affected their bargaining powers.

On a wider scale, Faugier (1996) found that the majority of the male clients had regular sexual partners, either wives or live-in partners, with whom they did not use condoms and who were at obvious risk of infection from their activities. In addition, a relatively high number of bisexual men were having sexual contact with female prostitutes as well as a regular female partner and casual male partners. In the light of AIDS, these men seemed to represent a distinct group who, in terms of their sexual contacts, could be viewed as 'out of control' and constituting a major risk to male and female partners alike.

IMPACT OF SOCIAL MARGINALIZATION AND THE LAW AND ITS ENFORCEMENT

In the UK prostitution is not illegal, although of course living off a prostitute's earnings is. This ambiguous legal situation means that prostitution can supply the fast cash earnings required to purchase heroin or cocaine with little risk of a custodial sentence. Criminal sanctions are generally much lower than for property offences usually committed by male drug users. Perry (1991) points out that this state of affairs maintains the economic dependence of women and the dominance of men right into the fringes of illegal society: 'The woman's earning power is typically controlled by a "male protector" who may also be seen as responsible for initiating and maintaining her degradation.'

It is an offence for a man to solicit a prostitute from a motor vehicle (kerb-crawling), although the arrests of women for soliciting generally disproportionately outnumber the arrests of male clients. However, in addition to the risk of arrest and the legal and social consequences of exposure, clients often fall victim to robbery when having sex in cars in secluded places. The majority of male clients have homes, security and a reasonable disposable income, which is a far cry from the circumstances of the majority of street prostitutes, especially those involved with drugs. Fearful for their lives, and (more importantly to them) their reputation, marriage or job, most do not report the crime. Thus, within this context it is hardly surprising that clients remain an extremely secretive group (Faugier and Cranfield 1995).

Laws against prostitution inform our prejudices towards those who sell sex. In 1989, data from the New York State *Uniform Crime Report* showed that 11,951 adult women were arrested for being engaged in prostitution, as compared to only 632 male customers, and only 293 persons were arrested for pimping. These figures are representative of nationwide practices and reveal an overwhelming bias towards arrests of female prostitutes compared to male clients, and an extremely infrequent arrest pattern of men on pimping charges. McKeganey and Barnard (1992a) argue that there must be better ways of responding to prostitution, particularly in the light of AIDS, than enforced legal controls which, far from removing prostitution, serve to drive it further underground. Rio (1991) argues that none of the traditional goals of imposing criminal sanctions (i.e. punishment, deterrence and rehabilitation) are furthered by the current prohibition and explicates the advantages offered by a system of decriminalized or legalized prostitution. Rather than stigmatizing prostitutes and making them subject to further legal constraints, services in areas of risk management need to be developed for both prostitutes and their clients.

DISCUSSION

In his 1979 review of prostitution, Goldstein highlights reports concerning well-educated professional women exchanging sexual favours for professional or other services and refers to this as a 'single woman's survival tactics', claiming that there is no surprise in poor drug-using women with scarce economic resources employing the sale of sex as a means of getting their drug supply. For Jolin (1994), however, the issue is deeper and clearly related to gender relations in society and inherent profound cultural contradictions originating from the desire of men as the dominant social group to ensure promiscuity for themselves and chastity for women:

> Men want sex with different women and they want women to have sex only with one man, a theoretical impossibility to which men have found a practical, albeit controversial, solution, one that requires setting aside a few women to meet the demands of men without substantially reducing the availability of chaste women or threatening the chastity of wives.

In referring to these arrangements as the 'promiscuity-chastity-inequality' model of prostitution aetiology, Jolin argues that the term 'inequality' is employed to reflect men's social and economic dominance over women: 'As the model suggests, prostitution owes its existence to a sexual double standard, the implementation of which is predicated on the economic and social dominance of men over women.'

This sexual double standard has in turn created an ingrained perception that females, and in particular women who prostitute, are responsible for polluting males. Historical origins for these traditional beliefs are manifest as in Britain, where the Contagious Disease Acts of 1864, 1866 and 1869 defined venereal diseases as transmitted by women and forced them to undergo medical examinations to protect men's health. These acts portrayed the prostitutes as self-seeking and immoral whereas their clients were depicted as behaving naturally:

> There is no comparison to be made between prostitutes and the men who consort with them. With the one sex, the offence is committed as a matter of gain; with the other, it is an irregular indulgence of a natural impulse.
>
> (Cited in Pateman 1988: 264, from the Report of the Royal Commission into the Contagious Disease Acts of 1864, 1866 and 1869)

It is therefore not surprising that over a century later, with the advent of the AIDS virus in the 1980s, prostitutes have again found themselves cast as scapegoats for transmitting the virus to men. This assumption, however, has failed to be supported by research on the relationships between prostitutes, their clients and HIV risk behaviour, the results of which have been unclear, the only significant association being linked to drug use (Nichols 1989). In addition, the labelling of 'females as polluting' and 'males as victims' fails to address the fact that someone is passing the virus onto the prostitutes themselves in the first place: '*someone* who may be transmitting the virus to wives and girlfriends at the same rate' (Sacks 1996: 64). This has led to the role of their male clients, boyfriends and pimps being neglected.

Whereas female prostitutes have traditionally been seen as an important group in the transmission of HIV, their male clients have been disregarded either as a subject of health promotion or for research purposes. The shame and social stigma attached to being a prostitute, and being a client of one, currently acts as a powerful disincentive against men seeking guidance or counselling. Male clients are potential carriers not only of HIV but of many other sexually transmitted diseases to both sex workers and their other sex partners and they wield considerable power in the decision-making process in relation to safer sex (Leonard 1990). Evidence of continuing requests from clients for unsafe sex strongly suggests the need for campaigns targeted at clients, supported by services aimed at contacting clients and stressing the risks of unprotected sexual contact (McKeganey and Barnard 1992a: 87). Male clients must be acknowledged to be priority groups for AIDS education and prevention, and health information should be devised and delivered to clients as a matter of urgency, with the prime focus being more extensive condom use (Morgan Thomas 1990). In addition, research has shown that prevention strategies need to be directed as much at prostitutes' private lives with their private partners as they are at their work (Day and Ward 1990).

The sex industry is extensive and those who sell sexual services are vastly outnumbered by those who buy services; however there has been a noticeable lack of interest in men's roles, particularly that of clients. The apparent dearth of current literature available on these roles highlights the importance of more detailed research to explore clients' perceptions of HIV risk and the barriers to their wider use of condoms. Sexual partners of female prostitutes, and specifically male clients, constitute a very important group requiring far greater emphasis both in terms of epidemiological study and health promotion than has previously been the case.

Part IV

Health issues

Chapter 7

Health care and regulation

New perspectives

Helen Ward and Sophie Day

INTRODUCTION

> Alison was 16 when we first met. She was referred to us by a social worker because she was already known to be HIV positive. She had been working as a prostitute for at least three years, and thought she had got HIV from a boyfriend who was also positive. Over the next six years we saw a lot of her. She began to inject drugs regularly, continued to work as a prostitute and spent time in prison for petty crimes. After a few years she became depressed and worried about her illness, and then developed AIDS.

> Danielle was in her mid-30s when she began using the project clinic. She made a relatively good living from her work as a prostitute. She had drifted into prostitution and continued to work to support her daughter after she left her husband. We got to know her very well, seeing each other regularly over a period of seven years. Generally we met in the clinic, where she came for monthly check-ups even though she rarely had any problems. She was an 'ideal' consumer of health services and advice as she was extremely concerned about HIV. During our last meeting she explained how she was still looking for alternative 'straight' jobs, but the money was not good enough. She was killed by her boyfriend.[1]

We set up the Praed Street Project in 1986 to look at risks of HIV and other sexually transmitted disease in women working as prostitutes. We combined epidemiological and anthropological research with the development of a clinic and other services for prostitutes. When we completed our research in 1992, the prevalence of HIV infection had not changed, remaining around 1 per cent (Day *et al.* 1988; Ward *et al.* 1993).

Our research was based on a cohort of women who were followed for up to seven years. During that time our perspectives on research and the development of services became much broader. Four women died during the last two years. Two had AIDS; both were infected when they joined our study, one through injecting drug use and the other probably through heterosexual contact with an infected non-paying partner. The other two women did not have HIV; they were both murdered.

These deaths are reported as a reminder that AIDS is only one of many issues facing the women. They presented with other health problems: sexually transmitted infections, recurrent problems such as thrush or cystitis, concerns about fertility and infertility, psychological problems and physical injuries. Health issues were themselves raised in relation to wider concerns about money, housing, conditions at work, police, family, relationships, violence at work and at home.

Through developing the Praed Street Project we attempted to address some of these broader concerns, providing a range of services that go far beyond those normally associated with genitourinary medicine and sexual health. Many other projects across the country have faced the same issues and, like the Praed Street Project, are now under threat as specific AIDS budgets are withdrawn and health authorities and clinics are likely to focus narrowly on HIV prevention for those at highest risk – which at the moment does not include prostitute women.

This chapter is primarily a history of the Praed Street Project, of the people who worked in it and of those who used it, with the aim of elucidating different perspectives on our work. We start with a brief discussion of prostitution and the risks of HIV and other sexually transmitted diseases as a background to our work.

PROSTITUTION AND THE RISK OF HIV AND OTHER SEXUALLY TRANSMITTED INFECTIONS

There are no routine data on the numbers of prostitutes with HIV infection or other sexually transmitted diseases in the UK. Many reports in the press assume a high rate of infection. In 1992 two major newspapers carried a report that 75 per cent of prostitutes working in the King's Cross area of London had HIV (Delgado 1992; *Sunday Express* 1992). The source of this information was the local vice squad, who reportedly keep records of the presumed HIV status of the women on the national police computer, in addition to having pictures of all the 'infected' women on their notice board (Ward and Day 1992). Women might be added to the HIV list if another person tells the police that she may be infected. The high rates reported are likely to reflect police prejudice against prostitutes rather than the true level of infection.

To counter such uninformed speculation, there are estimates of the prevalence of HIV in prostitutes from a number of research projects in the UK. In Glasgow in 1991, 2.5 per cent of women working as prostitutes were infected with HIV; in Sheffield no women were infected (1986–7) and in Edinburgh 14 per cent of prostitutes had HIV infection in 1988 (Woolley *et al.* 1988; Thomas *et al.* 1990; McKeganey *et al.* 1992). The higher prevalence in Edinburgh reflects the inclusion of male sex workers in the sample and the local epidemic of HIV in injecting drug users. In our study, the small number of cases of HIV in prostitutes (1.7 per cent in 1986–8, 0.9 per cent in 1989–91) were related to either injecting drug use, or sex with a non-paying partner known to have HIV (Barton *et al.* 1987; Day *et al.* 1988; Ward *et al.* 1993).

In the UK as elsewhere in Europe and North America, prostitute women with a history of injecting drugs are at highest risk of HIV (Krogsgard *et al.* 1986; Centres for Disease Control 1987; Smith and Smith 1987; van den Hoek and van Haastrecht 1988; European Working Group 1993). The overlap between injecting drug use and prostitution varies by town and sector of prostitution. In London between 8 per cent and 14 per cent of women prostitutes reported ever injecting drugs, in Edinburgh 28 per cent and in Glasgow 71 per cent (Day *et al.* 1988; Woolley *et al.* 1988; Thomas *et al.* 1990; Ward *et al.* 1993). The variation is partly explained by the different ways women were recruited to the studies – the Glasgow sample was of street workers in an area where injecting was known to be common, whereas in London we recruited women working in a range of sectors of prostitution.

Prostitute women who inject drugs and share equipment are clearly at increased risk of HIV infection in the same way as other drug injectors. Prostitutes who do not inject may also be at increased risk because of their sexual contacts – either with clients or non-paying partners. This risk can be reduced by the consistent use of condoms, or by avoiding penetrative sex. Most studies in the UK have concluded that prostitutes now use condoms all or most of the time with their clients, and this is likely to be an important explanation for their relatively low rates of HIV.

In London, we found that the proportion of women reporting always using condoms with their clients for vaginal sex increased considerably over the years. In 1985 slightly less than 50 per cent of women said they used condoms with all clients for vaginal intercourse; by 1990 this had risen to 98 per cent. However, condom use with non-paying partners remained less common, and women are at risk of sexually transmitted infections from these men (Ward *et al.* 1993).

The various studies in the UK therefore suggest the following general picture in relation to HIV risk: women working as prostitutes report high levels of condom use in commercial sex, but remain at some risk of HIV from injecting drug use and from unprotected sex with non-paying partners. At present these two factors have not led to high levels of HIV infection. However, these women are at risk of other sexually transmitted infections, including gonorrhoea and chlamydia which are themselves associated with considerable morbidity. In London, 44 per cent of women interviewed in 1989–91 reported a past history of gonorrhoea (Ward *et al.* 1993). In Sheffield 28 per cent of sixty-eight women had at least one episode of gonorrhoea during 1986–7; 24 per cent had chlamydia (Woolley *et al.* 1988).

Concern about the risk of infection in women who work as prostitutes is not new. Attempts to control sexually transmitted diseases have often focused on prostitutes who are seen as a 'reservoir' of infection. Traditional epidemiology of sexually transmitted infections suggests the existence of a 'core group' of people, including prostitutes, who have a high prevalence of infection. The group then sustains sexually transmitted infection in the rest of the population (Brunham 1991). This epidemlological model is relatively crude, and does not explain the high variability in risks of infection in different populations, but it has nevertheless underpinned a lot of interventions. Infection control strategies frequently focus on this notional core group (Plummer *et al.* 1991).

This approach has often led to legal and social efforts to control prostitutes themselves rather than to control sexually transmitted disease. In the nineteenth century, for example, much of the legislation on venereal disease control was directed at inspecting prostitutes, denying them liberty if they were thought to be infected (Walkowitz 1980). In the UK, laws explicitly targeting prostitutes for compulsory examination were repealed, but the regulation of prostitutes still forms the basis of control programmes for sexually transmitted diseases in many countries. In Greece prostitutes are supposed to be registered with the police, and are required to attend a clinic twice a week for a stamp in their card to prove they are free from infection. Similar controls are found in parts of Austria and Germany (EUROPAP 1995).

In the 1980s, the debate about approaches to the control of HIV infection brought the issue of prostitution to the fore in many countries. By the mid-1980s there was fear that HIV would infect everyone who had multiple sexual partners, including prostitutes. This was reinforced by reports from different parts of the world where a high prevalence of HIV had been found in prostitute women. In 1985, researchers in Rwanda reported that over 80 per cent of prostitutes were infected with HIV (Van de Perre 1985). In Nairobi, the prevalence of HIV-I in prostitutes rose from 4 per cent in 1981 to 61 per cent in 1985 (Piot *et al.* 1987). In the USA, the prevalence of HIV ranged from zero in Nevada to 45.3 per cent in New Jersey (Centres for Disease Control 1987). In Amsterdam 35.4 per cent of 96 prostitutes were found to be infected (van den Hoek and van Haastrecht 1988).

While these reports may have hit the headlines, contrasting reports of a low prevalence of HIV among prostitutes came from other parts of Europe, North America and Africa (Neequaya *et al.* 1986; Centres for Disease Control 1987; Day *et al.* 1988; van den Hoek and van Haastrecht 1988).

It was wrong to assume, as many people did, that prostitution would confer the same risks of HIV in all places, or even that prostitution itself was comparable in different settings in the same country, or even city (Day 1988). The varied reports indicated that risks of HIV infection would vary widely between different groups of prostitutes, and this would reflect wider aspects of the epidemic, such as the degree of heterosexual transmission, along with the local conditions for prostitutes, including the degree of control over their working conditions, access to health care and the availability of condoms. The degree to which prostitution is associated with drug use and trade, which will itself depend on the history of prostitution locally, will influence HIV risk. Associations between prostitution and organized crime, notably the marketing of illicit drugs, have been documented from the early twentieth century to today (Allen 1984; Perkins and Bennett 1985).

It is clear that the risk of HIV infection, as with other sexually transmitted infections, varies widely (Ward and Day 1991). Strategies for reducing this risk must also be flexible. The work described in the rest of this chapter was our response to this challenge, through an attempt to understand health risks encountered by prostitutes and to identify strategies for minimizing these risks. At the end of the chapter, we discuss whether this has provided a more effective and acceptable approach than the standard public health interventions which see prostitutes as a reservoir of infection that needs to be controlled and cleansed.

A HISTORY OF THE PRAED STREET PROJECT

In the mid-1980s the likely impact of AIDS on different sections of the population was unclear, and initiatives emerged all over the country to try and reduce the spread of HIV. At St Mary's Hospital in London the genito-urinary medicine clinic already provided services for a number of prostitutes who were expressing concern about their risks of AIDS. We developed research to explore risks of HIV among prostitutes and, where relevant, methods to reduce this risk.

In 1986, Sophie Day began work as an anthropologist, supported by AVERT (the AIDS Virus Education and Research Trust). Helen Ward was working as a research doctor and already saw some prostitutes who used the clinic. After a few months, we developed a single research and service project, as described below, and in 1988 Helen Ward obtained support from the Medical Research Council to develop her research in an epidemiological direction.

We established specific clinic sessions for prostitutes, which later became known as the Praed Street Project clinic. It was a specialized service within the main genito-urinary medicine clinic. Women were able to make appointments to see the same staff, in contrast to the routine genito-urinary medicine clinic which operated on a walk-in basis with more than a dozen doctors. After attending the Praed Street Project clinic, women no longer had to explain or conceal their concerns.

The clinical service provided diagnosis and treatment of sexually transmitted infections, screening for HIV and cervical cancer, hepatitis B vaccination, advice on risk reduction and a range of referrals. From its inception, this clinic was linked to our research. A clinic that was useful to participants seemed an effective way of maintaining contact with women over time and, thus, establishing a cohort study. We conducted repeated interviews on a number of topics with women who returned monthly, or as frequently as they wanted, for a check-up.[2] In this way, we were able to collect longitudinal data on HIV and STD risks in relationship to their social context. These included data on individuals and their partnerships, including condom use, drug use and numbers of sexual partners, as well as material on institutions, such as sectors of the sex industry and the apparatus for policing prostitution.

During the first few months, we became familiar with women and their accounts of work, and attempted to understand 'sexual health' from their points of view. We learned (on both sides) what language to use and how to ask questions in an appropriate way as well as what answers to expect. With time, the cohort design allowed us to develop some rapport and to explore issues which we could not broach during a single interview, such as family, sexuality and money. We were able to trace careers in prostitution as women were followed up for a period of several months or years. The longitudinal data also allowed us to check the reliability of our questionnaires through repeat interviewing.

The research interviews were conducted in a way that placed emphasis on discussion of issues raised by the women themselves, rather than being confined to pre-set research questions. Interviews allowed for detailed discussion of risk reduction in response to specific situations described by the women, and frequently encompassed issues such as family, relationships, fertility, the law and money, which had important effects on the ability of women to practice prostitution safely. We were there to learn from the women about risk, and about what would be of use to them in terms of support and specific services. The Praed Street Project was then expanded and developed, as far as possible, in the direction indicated by participants.

The cohort provided a unique but by no means perfect framework for epidemiological and anthropological research. The cohort was not a random sample of all eligible women, there was a high rate of loss to follow-up and there was little information with which to investigate the consequent biases. However, we have incidence data on sexually transmitted diseases in those who did remain in follow-up, and can relate these to risk factors such as numbers of partners, types of sex and condom use.

As with the epidemiology, the study has both advantages and disadvantages from an anthropological perspective. We relied largely on interviews and conversations, many of which took place in the clinic. Nonetheless, we collected such data over a period of years with participants whom we knew well, sometimes for as long as eight years. And, with time, we came to know women not just as 'patients' but at their workplace and, indeed, at court; among groups of friends and colleagues.

This basic clinical service and combined research continued until 1988, when we began to expand the project. The Medical Research Council awarded a grant for a larger epidemiological study in which prostitutes would continue to be interviewed in the clinic but also in the community, through field-work linked to outreach. This grant allowed us to employ a research nurse, an interviewer and later a second doctor to assist in the provision of clinical services. The research nurse made the service more accessible for a number of women through greater flexibility and more time for formal and informal discussions. She was able to maintain personal contact with women, providing telephone help with booking appointments and reporting results (with the exception of HIV testing).

We also approached the Regional Health Authority (North West Thames) to fund an outreach worker to help us reach women who were not coming to the clinic. By 1988, in addition to those who presented to the genito-urinary medicine routine clinic, many new women were referred to us by friends and colleagues. This networking enabled us to meet women who might not have come to the general clinic, but it did not necessarily improve access to services for other women. The Regional Health Authority provided the funds for us to employ a worker for six months, initially to carry out an assessment of the need for outreach services, and second for premises (a Portakabin) where we could set up a drop-in centre.

With these additional resources we were able to expand the project considerably, both in research and services. The expanded research was not easy. We planned to enrol 200 women each year in a cross-sectional study to monitor trends in the prevalence of HIV infection, and to look more closely at the relationship between HIV and other sexually transmitted infections. We wanted to include women recruited through field work on the streets, in agencies, saunas, flats and other clinics in London. It took two years of hard work to recruit fewer than 300 women, and the majority of these were seen in the Praed Street Project clinic. Working outside of the clinic presented difficulties we had not fully anticipated, including the effect of heavy policing on the visibility of women working on the streets, fear of prosecution that made agencies and saunas reluctant to allow us onto their premises and the suspicions of women contacted by telephone about the nature of our work.

The same problems were found in relation to expanding the coverage of the services of the Project. We were concerned that the relatively low risk of HIV infection in women attending the Project clinic may have reflected the fact that these were the women who already had the best access to health care. Women with greater risks and less opportunity to make use of existing health services may have been missed by our services and research. We addressed these concerns through linking the research to the further development of services. If the services became more appropriate and accessible, the research would better reflect the situation of prostitutes in London; as the research improved, we would have a greater understanding of the women's concerns in relation to health and health care.

The development of the Praed Street Project from 1988 to 1991 related to three main areas: an expansion of the range of clinical services provided; the opening of a drop-in centre and the related provisions of non-medical advice and support services; and outreach work to make contact with women outside of the clinic.

CLINICAL SERVICES

The Praed Street Project was based within a genito-urinary medicine clinic, but the diagnosis and treatment of sexually transmitted infections formed only a small part of our work. During the first seven years of the project, detailed records were kept of nearly 2,842 clinic visits made by 462 women. Women complained of symptoms on about half of the visits, at other times they requested screening for sexually transmitted diseases, cervical cancer, hepatitis B and HIV infection. In addition, advice was sought on contraception and fertility, general-health issues, and for psychological and social problems. Women frequently attended for reassurance following condom failures, reported on almost one-third of the visits, or in relation to other situations where they were concerned about having exposed themselves to risks of infection.

Most genito-urinary medicine clinics are relatively limited in the range of medical services they offer, but these are constantly under pressure from patients to expand, providing wider services for people who prefer the confidentiality which they feel is lacking in general practice. This has motivated many gay men to try and use genito-urinary medicine clinics as their source of primary care, particularly in relation to HIV disease. A similar pattern occurred with some of the women we saw. We therefore expanded the clinical service to provide more general health care – women would present with complaints such as sore throats, chest infections, minor injuries and skin problems. Sometimes this reflected poor access to local health services – one-third reported that they were not registered with a GP, and 11 per cent worked but did not live in London. On other occasions it related to problems of identity. It is difficult for a woman to disclose her work to a GP, who may be her family and children's doctor, but the health problem may be related to work. A sore throat may be associated with oral sex. An injury may be work-related. A skin problem may create problems for work in the future. Reluctance to consult other health care professionals also reflected stigmatization and actual, or anticipated, rejection.

One woman came to the clinic requesting a referral for infertility treatment. She did not want to go to the local hospital as she had been there before. On a ward round a doctor had introduced her to his students as a prostitute, whose infertility problems were assumed to be obvious from this label. This woman, like several others, had been refused infertility treatment because she was considered 'unsuitable'. In response we attempted to set up referral networks to agencies and professionals whom we were confident would not react in this way.

Where appropriate we provided basic primary care for women in the clinic, or referred them to appropriate specialists. It was not always easy to respond. One of the most obvious and frequent needs was for contraceptive services. Prostitutes are not alone in finding the existing provision of sexual health services in the UK sometimes difficult to fathom (Queen *et al.* 1991). Genito-urinary medicine clinics provide screening for sexually transmitted diseases, HIV testing and counselling, cervical screening and diagnosis through colposcopy. Some also provide services for people with sexual problems. They do not in general provide contraceptive services such as prescribing the pill, fitting caps and coils. They may provide condoms, but for prevention of infection rather than prevention of pregnancy.

Family planning clinics on the other hand provide the full range of contraceptive services, also offer cervical screening, but are rarely able to carry out screening for and treatment of sexually transmitted infections. Both clinics may, or may not, offer referrals for termination of pregnancy. General practitioners provide a variable combination of the above services.

Between 1986 and 1989, we were unable to offer contraceptive services to women using the clinic, other than basic advice, referral to the local family planning clinic, and condoms. Initially even the condoms had to be obtained specifically for the project, through a combination of donations (from condom manufacturers) and research funding. Obstacles to developing the contraceptive services included territorial disputes between the disciplines of genito-urinary medicine and family planning, and, centrally, funding. Contraceptive services were funded separately from genito-urinary medicine. We eventually convinced the local district health authority and clinic management that this was a short-sighted policy, and basic contraceptive services were made available – but only to prostitutes using the Praed Street Project clinic, and to women with HIV infection. Other women using the routine genito-urinary medicine clinic still have to be referred elsewhere for anything other than emergency contraception. Once the contraceptive services were made available they became very popular with prostitutes and made up a steadily increasing part of the workload, accounting for approximately 10 per cent of Praed Street Project clinic visits in 1991.

Many women requested help and professional counselling, with work and other problems including relationships, drug use, depression and abuse. But there is a widespread lack of trust by women in prostitution of other professions. Social workers are feared most of all, but others, including doctors, health advisers and psychologists, are also threatening. Women expect, and their fears are all too often confirmed, a prejudiced and unhelpful response. Even the best professionals are likely to be insensitive to many specific issues facing prostitutes. To overcome this we initially offered some counselling within the Project, and set up *ad hoc* referral mechanisms to psychologists and counsellors we trusted. Later, we were able to offer more counselling within the Project, using outreach workers who were undergoing formal training and supervision.

From 1986 to 1992 the Praed Street Project clinic was open for around five half days a week. Women made regular appointments for a check up, or contacted us with specific queries relating to, for example, burst condoms, symptoms, pregnancy or requests for emergency contraception. Women taking part in the research would also be interviewed at each clinic visit, if there was time and it was appropriate. Interviews and conversations during the clinic interviews provided important data for the research, helping us to understand how risks of HIV and sexually transmitted infections were located, and dealt with, in relation to other concerns. Women talked of their work, the methods they used to reduce risks of infection, the impact of the law on their ability to work safely, personal relationships and family.

Health problems were often inseparable from other concerns. Pauline was worried about infertility. She described a miscarriage the previous year at the age of 17, and had not used contraception with her boyfriend since then but was still not pregnant. The pregnancy had been the result of a rape, the miscarriage blamed on an assault by her boyfriend. She began working on the streets after the miscarriage, but felt that the threat of being infertile meant it was not worth it. She was concerned to find out if she could still get pregnant, worried that an episode of gonorrhoea may have blocked her tubes. A year later, she came in and was found to be pregnant by her boyfriend. Three months later we saw her after a termination, which her parents had pressured her into having. A year later she was pregnant again, and considering another abortion. Pauline related her concerns about infertility to her work as a prostitute – as long as she continued to work she was unable to construct a 'straight' life where she might have a baby. A few years later she had stopped work and was planning to get married – she had met an older man who had 'rescued' her from prostitution and with whom she planned to start a family. The last time we met she was retreating from the idea of marriage and of having a baby with him, fearing that she would be trapped as a housewife. It appeared that once she had stopped working, fertility and having a child had become less dominant concerns.

Many women expressed similar concerns about infertility,

frequently in relation to future pregnancies rather than wanting a baby at the time, while others wanted a child immediately. Sandra was in her mid-20s and had been working for 18 months. She definitely wanted children, and described 'being at the stage of total paranoia at not being able to conceive'. Her fears about infertility related to past infections; 'funnily enough I've been cleaner in my working life than before. I had gonorrhoea, chlamydia and trichomonas when I had lots of boyfriends'. She used condoms, a natural sponge and spermicidal pessaries with all clients. Three years later we saw her with her 18-month-old son and she was delighted to be pregnant again. She was still working and requested a check up, concerned about getting an infection that might 'rot the baby'. Throughout this time Sandra had problems with a violent boyfriend, the father of her children. She went into deep depressions, and was referred for counselling, which she found helpful. She stopped regular visits to the Project after her first baby was born, and used other services, although she was still seeing some clients. She has since completed a training programme and has a job.

Through developing the range of services on offer, the Project clinic met different needs for women working in prostitution. For some women it provided their only contact with medical care, for others it was one of a selection of providers of health care. Some attended private doctors for check ups and specialist care, some used drug treatment agencies, some consulted private doctors to obtain slimming tablets. Many women described other activities related to improving their general health and fitness, including running, swimming, aerobics and weight training. Women used complementary health care such as osteopathy, reflexology and aromatherapy, and some had cosmetic surgery.

Through the clinic we learned how prostitutes avoided infections at work, advice which we could in turn pass onto other women. The basic advice we offered was to use condoms for vaginal, oral and anal intercourse, and to ensure that there was no contact prior to putting on the condom. Women made us aware of problems of condom use in oral sex, including pointing out that lipstick, oil based, could weaken the condom. We heard advice about how to encourage men to use condoms, through developing negotiating skills and practical skills in applying the condom.

Several other methods of trying to reduce risks were described. Jenny told us how she used a contraceptive sponge, one or more spermicidal pessaries and was considering using two condoms with each client for vaginal sex. We saw Susan twice in 1986, and at one visit we discussed whether or not she needed a throat swab to check for gonorrhoea. She explained that if a client did come in her mouth, she would gulp down Listerine and spit out the semen. She preferred to do oral as she felt she could make them come quicker. If she had vaginal sex during a period she would douche, and then use a diaphragm and spermicidal cream.

The women we saw described using spermicidal preparations as additional protection from infection long before it was being advocated by 'experts' as a possible way of reducing HIV transmission. Prostitutes were also the first to express fears about the safety of using the chemicals contained in spermicides and condom lubricants – concerns that are now the subject of extensive research and debate (Elias and Heise 1994; Weir *et al.* 1995; Ward *et al.* in press).

DROP-IN CENTRE

In 1988 we established Project offices separate from the main genito-urinary medicine clinic and opened a drop-in centre. The Praed Street Project clinic was still within the main clinic building. We first had a Portakabin in the car park below the clinic, next door to the Wharfside clinic, also a Portakabin, where HIV and AIDS out-patient clinics were based. This physical location added to our identity as 'outsiders', not fully part of the clinic and its more traditional services. But there were many advantages in this slight separation. Women did not have to enter the main building to visit us and check out what we were offering them. Women could come in for informal discussions, collect condoms, be interviewed, make appointments for the clinic or simply meet other women over tea and coffee. This took some months to attract women but subsequently became very popular.

After several months the main clinic moved into new premises (the Jefferiss Wing Clinic) and we moved the offices and drop-in to another part of the hospital. It was not easy to identify such premises and obtain permission to use them – we were funded through research money and employed through the medical school, not the hospital. It was the District Public Health Department that finally agreed to provide us with the premises within the hospital grounds. The new premises were a great improvement. We had three floors of a narrow old building; one became the meeting room and drop-in, the other two were offices. The drop-in was open for particular sessions, but many women dropped in at other times for a chat, advice or to pick up condoms. Recurrent themes emerged and led to the development of specific forms of advice and support.

Legal problems were commonly discussed by individuals and groups of women. These related to problems with the police and courts over repeated fines, and specifically in relation to arrests when not working. Women find it difficult to contest a prostitution-related charge when they have a record because the evidence required to obtain a conviction is so minimal. Prostitutes have many other legal problems related to the criminalization of their work – the difficulties in establishing legitimate businesses and incomes lead to problems with tax, mortgages and other loans. Property may be held by others to avoid some legal problems, but this produces other difficulties when that other person, frequently a boyfriend, reneges on the agreement. We contacted a legal organization, Release, to provide advice sessions in the drop-in centre.

Women turned to us for help when they faced various crises and found it difficult to gain access to other sources of support, such as social services. We responded through providing advice on welfare and housing issues (informally at first, but later using trained staff), and establishing formal links with other agencies who could provide practical help.

Through opening a drop-in centre the Project established a distinct identity beyond that of the individual staff who provided particular services. Prostitutes became users of the Praed Street Project rather than 'patients' or 'interviewees'. A drop-in centre can transform relations between staff and users. The relationship between health worker and prostitute in clinic consultations, interviews and one-to-one counselling is unequal. However good the training and motivation of the staff, prostitutes are often, like other patients and clients of services, placed at a disadvantage. In a drop-in, where there may be several prostitutes and one or two members of staff, that relationship begins to change. The drop-in can create the conditions for Project users to collectively assert their positions and define their needs.

Some women clearly found it easier to discuss safer sex, problem clients and health concerns in the drop-in than in the clinic. Where possible the clinic doctor and nurse participated in the drop-in sessions in order to reduce the barrier between the two, but there remained some women who would attend the drop-in but would not use the clinic.

At the same time, the drop-in is not an appropriate place for other women. Some clinic attendees expressed horror at the idea of visiting the Project and drop-in, for fear of being seen there, meeting other women. Although they would likely meet other prostitutes in the waiting room of the Praed Street Project clinic, this was seen as less threatening to some women than being in a situation where they were together *as prostitutes*. For a project to meet the needs of all prostitutes, these differences between women need to be recognized and addressed.

The drop-in also served important functions for the staff working in the Praed Street Project. While it was often irritating to be interrupted in the middle of some work in order to answer the door to someone dropping in when the drop-in was 'closed', the informal contact with women in this situation was invaluable in terms of understanding their lives. In addition, the group drop-in sessions provided very positive feedback about the Project, and made us feel that the work was highly valued by users. This was a great strength at times when we felt rather less valued by other sections of the health service.

OUTREACH WORK

We began outreach work in 1988. As in the clinic, research work and service provision were integrated, and 'field-work' was carried out at the same time as taking services out into the community. An outreach worker was employed to develop this work, specifically looking at health needs of women met in settings other than the clinic.

From 1989 to 1992 fieldwork and outreach took place on the streets of west, north and east London, in the magistrate's courts and in saunas, escort agencies and flats in west London. The aim was to find women working as prostitutes, to offer them condoms and health information, advertise the services available at the Praed Street Project, and to ask them about their work and health. Through this work we hoped to improve their access to services (at St Mary's and elsewhere), and to find out whether our research findings from the clinic were more widely applicable.

Street outreach was made difficult by persistent heavy policing in west London. The main effect of the heavy policing – designed to reduce the visibility of prostitution in the area – was to make women difficult to find, and to make them reluctant to talk to us for fear of becoming more 'visible'. We contacted the local police to inform them of our work and to seek some assurance that they would not use talking to us as evidence that women were working. We received a verbal guarantee to this effect, but it was not always respected in practice by the police on the street.

Information collected during outreach was not standardized. Some women would talk to us for some time, and we would meet them repeatedly, others would be seen only transiently. Information was recorded from talking to sixty-two different women during the first few months of street outreach. Twelve (19 per cent) were already using the St Mary's genito-urinary medicine clinic – five of whom used the Project clinic, while seven used the general clinic without disclosing their work. Five more used other clinics, and six used local drugs services. Shortly after the outreach, a further ten women (16 per cent) made use of the Praed Street Project services.

This street work showed that while some women were already in contact with genito-urinary medical services, only a minority used them regularly, and many did not disclose their work. But discussions revealed that access to genito-urinary medical services was not necessarily the primary issue. A quarter of the women described problems with drug use, some of whom wanted needle exchange and other drug services which we were not able to provide. The other major request for advice related to reproduction: four women were pregnant and receiving no antenatal care; two described recent miscarriages, both related to violence; four other women described problems of conceiving and wanted fertility investigations. A range of other untreated health needs were described: two were worried about CIN, and two had never had smears; one wanted to come for an 'AIDS test', reporting that she had been refused one at another London hospital.

Several women reported pelvic problems. One said she had 'stomach pains' and subsequently attended for a check-up. A second woman suspected a pelvic infection while a third reported an untreated infection which had been diagnosed in prison. A fourth knew she had chronic pelvic inflammatory disease but had no GP or other health care. One woman thought she had a 'dose' (gonorrhoea). One said she was bleeding badly. One reported a vaginal discharge. Two wanted check-ups, as they had not attended clinics recently, in one case for sixteen years. A few women reported current treatment for their health; one woman was being treated for a cyst and another was receiving antenatal care.

Health needs were not easily distinguished from other aspects of street prostitution. Two women were worried about their children and the law. One, for example, wanted access to her child in the care of her mother. Two wondered about their rights on arrest as they were under-age; they were particularly worried that they might be sent home. Four women were currently suffering the effects of work-related violence (stitches, bruises, breakages, rape).

The above figures do not fully illustrate the range of health needs reported by prostitutes, nor the importance of field-work as a service in its own right as well as a means of accessing women to other health services. Many women took advantage of our visits to discuss health issues. In general, these issues were contextualized by reference to policing and the law on the one hand, and problems of safety with clients on the other. At times, health issues were also related to the difficulties of making a living. Much of our data on health were acquired gradually, after several meetings, as shown by a single illustration, concerning a woman, 'Christine', whom we met eight times.

> The second time I met Christine, she described how she had been raped and beaten the previous month on the 'beat' (the street area where she worked). She attended St Mary's STD clinic, under her real (that is, legal) name, and she told neither the doctor nor the health adviser the circumstances of this rape. She did not describe her work. Because she had used her 'real' name, she did not report the rape to the police: she did not want her name revealed in court.
>
> Two weeks later, Christine had been attacked by a man with a knife. She was not hurt. The police had arrived, but they 'just let the guy walk off'. At this meeting, Christine also described three past pregnancies, the first was a stillbirth, the second lived for 10 minutes and the third miscarried at 7 months. She had been told that she would not be able to have children and requested further investigations into her reproductive health.

> At our third meeting, three weeks later, Christine was preoccupied. She had been sent a routine letter from St Mary's STD clinic. This had been opened by another woman and everyone was gossiping about what infection Christine might have. Christine was still suffering from the rape. Her GP 'simply prescribed sleeping pills'. A doctor at St Mary's STD clinic offered 'only an HIV test'. Subsequently, Christine made use of the PSP doctor and drop-in.
>
> At our eighth meeting, Christine was particularly concerned about policing in relation to her health. She had been arrested on the way to a video shop and kept in a cell all night, where she had suffered an asthma attack.

In summary, the street work identified a significant number of women who were not using our, or any other, service and yet revealed that they had considerable health care needs. The outreach succeeded in establishing contact, and some of these women later used the Praed Street Project drop-in and clinic. In addition to the ten mentioned above, more subsequently attended, but in some cases it was many months or years later. On outreach we could deal directly with some of the problems raised – providing information on infections and explaining how to register for antenatal care, for example. We were unable to follow most of these women up to see whether or not they did contact appropriate services because of the changing conditions on the street. Sustained heavy policing made it difficult for us as well as the women, and contacts were lost.

Magistrates' Courts are another useful place to meet women working as prostitutes – they usually appear before the court in the morning after being charged with prostitution-related offences the previous night. During 1990 and 1991 project workers made 115 visits to four London courts, and made 216 contacts with 119 different women. As on the street outreach, women were given condoms and information about the clinic; unlike the night-time outreach it was sometimes possible for project workers to bring women met in court directly to PSP if they needed medical or other services urgently. Thirty-five women met through the courts agreed to an interview for our research project. This work also brought us into contact with a number of male prostitutes. While PSP services were specifically for women, we could refer these men to other services (such as the Working Men's Project and Streetwise).

Women working from their own premises were contacted on the phone by research workers and by a PSP participant who had contacts with women working in flats who volunteered to do sessional work for the Project. The phone numbers are widely advertised in local telephone kiosks, contact magazines and local papers. This method was very labour intensive and rather frustrating, as many of the lines were disconnected, some women had several lines, and a few women did not want to talk to us.

We had more problems trying to contact women working in saunas, massage parlours and agencies. Unsolicited visits and phone calls generally met with hostility from the receptionists and management. This is not surprising, as these businesses are frequently approached by the police in different guises with the aim of bringing charges against them. Later on these attempts were more successful as we were able to use existing contacts met through the clinic or the drop in to introduce us into the saunas or agencies. Since 1992 this work has become much more systematic and is proving a successful way of making contact with women, particularly those who are new to the area.

PERSPECTIVES ON THE PRAED STREET PROJECT

In 1992 the various research projects came to an end. Attempts to secure continued funding from the Medical Research Council were unsuccessful because prostitutes were considered to be at insufficient risk of HIV to make continued follow-up valuable. By this time we had also completed a research project describing HIV risks in the clients and other male sexual partners of prostitutes, and were in the process of writing up the results of various aspects of the work. There was a danger that the Project would end with the research, something we were determined to avoid. We felt that a clear need had been established for this type of project, and that the Praed Street Project team were uniquely placed to do this in west London.

We took proposals to the hospital, and the district and regional health authorities. The District Health Authority agreed to fund the drop-in and outreach project as part of HIV services. The initial team was a project coordinator, two outreach workers and a part-time administrative worker (who was never appointed). All three had worked on the research project and were skilled in working in this field. The medical side of the project was funded half through research (for a study of the acceptability of spermicides in condom lubricants) and half through routine clinic services.

The services have developed further since the main research ended, including initiatives such as the provision of self-defence classes for women, building closer links with drug agencies, and a new research project has been set up to look at the particular needs of prostitutes who use crack.

The range of services provided and the explicit commitment to an holistic approach to health does not sit easily within the clinically-led hospital structure. The work of the Project is labour intensive – it may take several contacts with a woman on the streets or in the courts before she attends even the drop-in centre, and more work before she feels it appropriate to have a check-up, contraceptive advice and hepatitis B vaccination. Some women will attend the drop-in more or less weekly for months at a time, with no specific problem that requires intervention. To Project workers and users the need for this intensive and sustained work is clear. Over the years Project workers have seen women move from abusive situations where they were extremely vulnerable, to a position of greater stability and independence.

We first met one Project user, Suzanne, in 1988. She found it difficult to use the clinic due to a lack of confidence and mistrust. Through regular visits to the drop-in, interviews and counselling she began to open up about her problems. She was in an abusive relationship which led to visits when she was injured, frightened, angry; she also needed treatment for a number of sexually transmitted infections. At other times she was happy and optimistic, which we found difficult as we knew it was unlikely to be sustained. But after many years of contact with the Project, she has found a way of taking control. She is completing a university degree and looking for a new job, has left her abusive partner behind. It is impossible to say how much the Project contributes to such a process, but from her perspective at least, it provided a setting where she could find support through all kinds of crises, knowing that she would not be rejected, and indeed that she, and her views, were valued.

From the perspective of other people working in the health service, the level of individual and group support provided to women using the Project appears as a luxury, as it does not conform to standard clinical practice. But the justification for the service lies outside the realm of standard clinical care, where efficiency is measured in throughput of patients. The Praed Street Project has a broader aim than identifying and treating infections.

From the public health perspective, prostitutes are seen as having poor access to standard health care as a result of stigma and marginalization, and the Project aims to improve access, removing barriers to the use of clinics. This in turn is important as prostitutes are likely to be in greater need of input from the health services because they are potentially at high risk of acquiring, and transmitting, infections. Additional resources directed at prostitutes may therefore be justified from a public health (i.e. population) perspective. However, the more successful the Project is in reducing the risks of HIV and other infections, the less such a view appears to be valid. If prostitutes are not at a high risk, why fund special prevention projects?

The Praed Street Project is one of many that have been established over the last ten years, the majority with a specific focus on sexual health and HIV risk. As part of a European collaborative survey, we identified over eighty projects in the UK that work in whole or part with prostitutes on the issue of health (Casey *et al.* 1995). Most operate with a similar holistic approach to health and explicitly reject abolitionist or regulationist approaches to prostitution. Advice and services are provided in the framework of 'harm minimization' that became the dominant approach to health promotion in relation to HIV – the health workers' role is not to comment on behaviour itself (such as drug use, sexual orientation or prostitution) but to help reduce the health risks associated with such behaviours.

There is a dilemma facing all projects working in HIV and sexual health in the second half of the 1990s. AIDS money is no longer 'ring fenced', it is part of the general budgets. Many innovative projects, like the Praed Street Project, were initially established in response to AIDS, and funded with ear-marked money. Now this is going, projects are forced to justify their role in relation to NHS managers' and purchasers' perspectives – usually shrouded in terms like 'health gain'. Projects are asked to provide rapid evaluations of their work, to define outcome measures which can be related to input resources.

It should be clear from the description of the Project and the case studies outlined that such assessments are not easy. Outcomes, such as the ability to leave a violent partner, may take many years to achieve. Health gain is easy to measure in terms of numbers of infections treated, but it is very hard to estimate numbers of infections prevented in a group using such a project. Finding outcome measures for broad health and support projects is going to be difficult, but is a challenge we need to take up if much of this kind of work is to survive.

In 1992, we (HW and SD) left the Project and had to move on to other jobs and research projects. Initially we retained an official role as part of a management committee of the Project, but that was later disbanded. Since then we have continued to have informal links, and to be involved in specific research projects, including the study of condoms and spermicides, and recently on crack-cocaine use.

Leaving the Project was difficult, but the distance and time does enable us to reflect on the work. What is missing from the perspectives outlined above is that of the women working in prostitution. Project workers work hard, are stressed and insecure, but are convinced of the need for the work to continue. Planners and managers are not so convinced, and want hard data to convince them of the need to provide such supportive services for prostitutes. Public health workers may see the value in the preventive and holistic approach.

Prostitutes will not all have a similar view. Many, and certainly those who regularly use the services, think that they are very valuable and react angrily to any suggestion of cutting back on services. But other women may be suspicious of the projects, seeing them as reinforcing the idea that prostitutes need to be helped and are in some way passive or victims.

Cheryl Overs, from the International Committee on Prostitutes' Rights, questions the hundreds of projects in the world designed to 'educate prostitutes'. She warns:

> The funds are not directed at sex workers for their own sake, but because they are viewed as people particularly likely to infect others. . . . It is important not to misunderstand the nature of this benevolence – it has nothing to do with women's health, or the rights of prostitutes. There has been no change in policies or motivation, but rather these are pragmatic moves to protect the client. If prostitutes' rights were the priority, the focus of

> prevention efforts would be to improve working conditions to enable women to insist on condom use and to work in safety without fear of male violence, or to prevent them from being unwillingly dependent on the protection of other people or the police. Human rights would be the central issue, as this would lead to greater control over working conditions and greater self-esteem.
>
> (Overs 1994: 114–21)

It would be wrong to view all projects as the same, and many of the workers in them are concerned as much with self-esteem as they are with sexually transmitted diseases. Overs is right to remind us of the motives of many of those who fund these initiatives. But that should not blind us to the fact that many projects that have developed in response to AIDS have had beneficial effects for prostitutes. The distribution of free condoms, appropriate advice on safety at work, improved clinical services, access to sympathetic legal advice – all are valuable in their own right.

There is one further concern. Health promotion is often very worthy, but it can also be viewed as a form of social control. In relation to prostitution, health projects are concerned with promoting safer sex, to protect the woman and her client. At best, health promotion provides people with the ability to make informed choices. At worst it imposes a conformity whereby anyone who chooses not to be healthy is seen as deviant. Within prostitute projects this may have the effect of excluding some women from contact because they do not conform, because they take drugs or do not want to have regular check-ups, for example.

On the other side there is a danger of 'medicalizing' prostitutes. Recommending medical checks is crucial to diagnose asymptomatic infection, but there are dangers that this makes some women feel a great dependency, whereby they cannot be 'healthy' without the approval of a doctor. This form of medicalization may reduce rather than increase the control women have over their health.

A second, related, problem is that health issues have once again come to dominate much of the debate on prostitution. Those of us with an interest in the problems that prostitutes face have turned away from broader social aspects of prostitution towards the narrow concerns of a health promotion team. We have consequently tended to neglect the broader debates on prostitution, exploitation and stigma, except insofar as they have an impact on health issues.

The law, for example, is seen primarily as an obstacle to the effective delivery of health promotion messages and the ability of prostitutes to carry condoms, not as a systematic form of oppressing those who work in prostitution.

The last decade has seen a growth in 'experts' on prostitution. We are part of that phenomenon, and it is often tempting to speak out as advocates for the women we have worked with. To ensure that the interests and demands of prostitutes are not drowned by the focus on health, our 'expertise' needs to be balanced with, and challenged by, the voice of prostitutes themselves.

Chapter 8

Alcohol, drugs and social milieu

Martin Plant

INTRODUCTION

Since early times prostitution has frequently been associated with drinking and with other forms of drug use. Indeed, the locales in which sex is available for sale are often also places wherein alcohol or other psychoactive drugs may be imbibed, legally or illicitly. In many cultures pleasure-seeking and risk-taking commonly involve both sex and various forms of drug use. Moreover, there is an extensive literature linking sexual behaviour with the use of alcohol and other substances. In recent years the advent of HIV/AIDS has provided a stimulus to studies concerned with the possible connection between drinking or illicit drug use and high-risk sex. A number of these studies have focused on prostitutes and their clients as potentially being at special risk in this respect. This chapter examines some of the available evidence on this topic, with special reference to the situation in Britain. This evidence is placed in the general context of patterns of alcohol and drug use in society and of evidence on the connection between drinking and drug use in relation to high-risk sexual behaviour and the transmission of HIV/AIDS.

ALCOHOL AND DRUG USE IN BRITAIN

Humanity has long exhibited a great propensity to use psychoactive (mind-altering) drugs. Virtually every known society has tolerated, if not actively sanctioned or revered, some forms of recreational drug use. In addition, drugs are often also integrated into religious rites and major social events. Most adolescents and adults in Britain consume alcohol and an increasingly large proportion have also used illicit drugs such as cannabis. Tobacco use, though declining, continues to be widespread, especially amongst those in lower socioeconomic positions.

The role of alcohol in British culture is so deeply entrenched that the invitation to 'have a drink' is frequently assumed to indicate an alcoholic beverage. Evidence indicates that even young children begin to develop strong impressions about alcohol and that by adolescence, most people regard drinking as a hallmark of sociability and maturity (Davies and Stacey 1972; May 1992; Plant and Plant 1992; Fossey 1994). Surveys further indicate that amongst British teenagers and young adults, the overwhelming majority have begun to drink by the ages of 15 and 16. In England and Scotland as a whole only a small minority, 3–4 per cent appear to be abstainers at this age (Plant *et al.* 1990; Plant and Foster 1991). Even so it appears that in some areas, such as Northern Ireland and the Western Isles of Scotland, a substantial proportion of teenagers do not drink (Loretto 1994; Anderson and Plant in press). This probably reflects a number of cultural factors, including religion. The normality of alcohol consumption is emphasized by the findings of Foster *et al.* (1990) that 93 per cent of adult males and 88 per cent of females in Britain were classified as drinkers. Surveys suggest that the heaviest drinking sections of the community include young single males and females in their late teens and early 20s. Males generally drink more heavily than females and males are also more likely than females to experience adverse consequences (problems) because of their drinking (M.L. Plant, 1990; McDonald 1995). Most of those who drink do so in moderation and without evident harm. Even so, some people drink in ways that cause problems. The harm associated with heavy or inappropriate drinking includes medical, social and public disorder problems. There are occupational and regional variations in the levels of such problems. These reflect, amongst other factors, long-standing social and cultural differences in drinking habits and in the social pressures to drink.

The use of other psychoactive drugs is generally far more restricted than that of alcohol. Even so a substantial minority of people do use such substances. Tobacco smoking has been declining in the United Kingdom, as in a number of other countries. In 1974 it was reported that 45 per cent of those over the age of 16 in Britain smoked. By 1988 this proportion had fallen to 32 per cent. The prevalence of smoking varies by region, with the highest levels in Scotland, Wales and the North of England. Smoking is much more commonplace amongst those in lower socioeconomic positions than those in higher positions. A number of studies also indicate that smoking amongst teenagers in Britain is more prevalent amongst females than amongst males (Foster *et al.* 1990; Plant and Plant 1992). Tobacco use, like alcohol consumption patterns, varies according to occupational group. This fact has considerable relevance to the subject of this chapter, as will be elaborated below. In contrast to the decline in smoking, the use of illicit drugs has been increasingly markedly. Surveys suggest that in many areas of Britain at least a quarter of those in the age range 16–18 have at some time used such substances and that in some areas illicit drug use is far more widespread (Plant and Plant 1992; Loretto 1994; Anderson and Plant in press). One study, for example, indicated that 51 per cent of a study group of teenagers in the Manchester area had used illicit drugs (Parker *et al.* 1995). Most illicit drug use is confined to cannabis, although other substances are also used. Surveys of teenagers and young adults suggest that the majority of those who have used illicit substances have done so in only a very limited and often temporary way. Drug use is rare, but by no means uncommon, amongst pre-adolescents. Some studies have noted the use of glues and solvents by such individuals. Moreover, a number of drug workers and other commentators have reported some evidence of the increasing use of other drugs by children in London and other, mainly urban, areas. It is clear that there has been an increase in the use of substances such as heroin, cocaine, MDMA (ecstasy) and a variety of so called 'dance drugs'. Moreover drugs such as amphetamines, benzodiazepines and LSD have been in illicit circulation for over two decades and continue to be used recreationally by some individuals. There has been a steady rise in 'problem drug use', as indicted by statistics recording the numbers of 'addicts' notified by doctors. These have risen from 1,426 in 1970 to 33,952 in 1994. Convictions for drug offences have also risen. In 1979 14,339 persons were found guilty of drug offences. In 1993 75,122 people were dealt with for drug offences (Plant and Plant 1992; Home Office 1995a, 1995b).

ALCOHOL, DRUGS AND HIGH-RISK SEX

There is a rich folklore connecting sex and the use of alcohol or drugs. In Shakespeare's *Macbeth* it was stated that alcohol consumption 'provokes the desire but it takes away the performance'. Moreover, drinking, illicit drug use and sexuality have been linked for a variety of social, psychological reasons (Cavan 1966; Soloman and Andrews 1973; Ridlon 1988).

It is a well-established belief that consuming alcohol or using drugs such as cannabis, cocaine or amphetamines might lead to 'disinhibition' and thereby encourage potentially risky behaviours. 'Disinhibition' has been defined in several ways, but basically means the release of inclinations or behaviours that would otherwise be restrained or held in check. In many societies it is assumed that drinking alcohol, for example, leads to relaxation and makes it more likely that an individual will act in a carefree manner. Drinking has often been used as an excuse for behaviour that later provokes shame or regret: 'I would not have done it if I had been sober.' Available scientific evidence suggests that the role of alcohol in relation to disinhibition is complex. In fact the effects of any drug depend upon the chemistry of the substance, the characteristics of the user and the environment in which use occurs. Social setting and expectations are influential, even if they are very often difficult to assess (Bush 1980; Room and Collins 1983; Coles and Stokes 1985).

Clearly, the assumption that psychoactive drug use and sexual behaviour might be connected is long-standing. In spite of this, scientific interest in this topic has been greatly stimulated by concerns about the spread of HIV infection. From very early in the recorded history of HIV transmission, it was evident that the sharing of infected injecting equipment by intravenous drug users was an important factor (Strang and Stimson 1990).

A very influential study concluded that US gay men who had combined sex with drinking or the use of drugs such as cannabis were particularly likely to report having engaged in 'high-risk' behaviours (Stall *et al.* 1986). These findings prompted a flurry of research activity into the possible connection between drinking and the use of non-injected drugs and sexual risk-taking. These have been reviewed in detail elsewhere (Plant and Plant 1992; Leigh and Stall 1993; Plant 1993, 1996; World Health Organization 1994). Available evidence on this topic has been reported from the

USA, Britain. Australia and Norway. This indicates that amongst young adult heterosexuals those individuals who drink heavily are more inclined to engage in high-risk sex and a number of other potentially dangerous activities. The latter include smoking and illicit drug use. Some individuals clearly take more risks than do others. Studies of gay men have produced rather more inconsistent results in this respect, with only some concluding that heavier drinkers take more risks. One of the largest studies, from Britain, concluded that drinking was unrelated to sexual behaviour (Weatherburn 1994). Miller *et al.* (1995), examining results from two surveys of young adults, concluded that risk-taking was neither general nor specific. A number of types of risk-taking were evident. These included illicit drug use, heavy drinking and sexual risk-taking. Different patterns of association were evident amongst different sub-groups of people. The most striking feature of research into this topic is that not a single study of which this author is aware has demonstrated that consuming alcohol on a specific occasion does foster high-risk sex. Many people appear to believe, or at least to report, that there is such a connection, but it has not been born out empirically.

ALCOHOL, DRUGS AND PROSTITUTION

Prostitution is a world-wide activity involving enormous numbers of people. For the purposes of this chapter, 'prostitution' is defined as the provision of sexual services in exchange for some form of payment. Many of the men and women who work as prostitutes drink alcohol, smoke and use illicit drugs. In part this is simply a reflection of general social habits, especially those that relate to young adults. As noted above, both drinking and illicit drug use are commonplace amongst many social groups in Britain, and in many other countries. The relationship between drinking, drug-taking and prostitution is not straightforward. As noted above, different sub-groups of people use legal and illicit drugs in different ways. Habits vary between localities and even different groups within a single locality. This is true of both alcohol, the most widely used drug, and of tobacco and illicit drugs. Moreover, the links between drinking and drug use and prostitution are further influenced and complicated by the ways in which the sex industry is organized in specific localities and the ways in which services for problem drug users are arranged (Plant 1990). These influences are reflected by major differences between even neighbouring cities, such as Edinburgh and Glasgow. In Edinburgh there is relatively little street prostitution, while this is commonplace and extensive in Glasgow. If 'saunas' and 'massage parlours' are permitted in a town, this may provide relatively unobtrusive, safe and congenial working conditions for men and women who might otherwise meet clients by working around bars or on the streets. If a town has an efficient drug prescribing service this may reduce the necessity for 'problem drug users' or drug-dependent individuals to engage in prostitution in order to purchase drug supplies. In some localities, police policy simply does not permit widespread street prostitution. The latter is, in fact, illegal in the United Kingdom and in a number of other countries.

A series of studies have examined the connection between prostitution, alcohol consumption and illicit drug use. As noted above, such investigations have been greatly encouraged by the advent of HIV/AIDS and by its obvious link in some areas with intravenous drug use. A convincing body of evidence supports the conclusion that the occupational culture of the sex industry actively fosters the relatively heavy use of alcohol, tobacco and illicit drugs. The evidence supporting this view is now briefly presented.

An Edinburgh study elicited information from both male and female prostitutes (Morgan Thomas *et al.* 1989; Morgan Thomas 1990; Plant *et al.* 1990). This investigation collected information by interviewing a non-random study group of 102 males and 103 females. The mean age of the females was 26 and that of the males was 23. Only 4 per cent had stayed on at school beyond the age of 16, in comparison with 39 per cent of Scottish school pupils in general. This investigation showed that many of these mainly young working class men and women contacted clients in licensed premises and that many were very heavy drinkers. In addition, illicit drug use was commonplace. Even so, only a fifth of those interviewed reported ever having used drugs by injection. Females were more likely than the male prostitutes or 'rent-boys' to report intravenous drug use. A number of people commented that drug-dependent females are more likely than drug-dependent males to engage in prostitution to pay for drug supplies; males are more likely to engage in theft. The overall levels of psychoactive drug use reported by the Edinburgh prostitutes were high. A total of 87 per cent of females and 73 per cent of the males interviewed reported that they smoked. This is in contrast with only a third of adults in Britain as a whole, though the level of smoking is highest amongst manual/blue-collar workers (Foster *et al.* 1990). As noted above, heavy drinking was commonplace amongst this study group. Only eight females and six males indicated that they did not drink. Approximately two-thirds of the study group reported having been intoxicated during the week preceding interview. Amongst those who had drunk in the past week, the mean alcohol consumption for the females was 48.1 units and that for males was 63.8 units. A 'unit' is equivalent to half a pint of normal strength beer, lager, cider or stout or to a single bar-room measure of spirits or to a glass of wine. Respondents were also asked how much they had consumed on their most recent drinking occasion, not necessarily in the past week. Female drinkers reported a mean consumption of 13.9 units and males a mean of 17.7 units. In comparison with studies of both the general population and of other young adults, these people included many very heavy drinkers. It should be noted that Edinburgh does not have a major 'red-light area' and that most prostitute–client contacts are conducted indoors. Many initial contacts are made in bars, discos and other similar venues in which drinking is a prominent, if often only a secondary, social activity. Under such circumstances, drinking and smoking were strongly encouraged. The vast majority of respondents also reported having used cannabis: 90 per cent of males and 83 per cent of females had smoked cannabis and more than half had done so in the month before interview. In addition a minority had used other substances such as amphetamines, LSD, benzodiazepines, glues and solvents. Only a minority, it should be noted, had used drugs other than cannabis in the past month. A third of the females and eleven males had at some time used heroin. Cocaine had been used by 48 females and 28 males. Females were also more likely than males to report having used benzodiazepines (such as Librium, Valium, Temazepam and Ativan).

Forty-one individuals, roughly 20 per cent of those interviewed, stated that they had used drugs by injection. Fewer than a third of those who reported being current injectors stated that they had never shared injecting equipment with other people. All of the injectors noted that they had shared equipment in the past. Morgan Thomas (1990: 100) concluded:

> The remaining seventeen respondents who currently used intravenous drugs and who still shared their injecting equipment were asked about the frequency with which they did so. The five males reported sharing equipment on average five times per month with an average of 2.3 people. The twelve females reported sharing on average 7.5 times per month with an average of 6.3 people. Their sharing was not confined to Edinburgh. Three males and nine females reported sharing in other parts of the UK.

This Edinburgh study indicated that approximately half of the male and female prostitutes interviewed reported having experienced some form of adverse consequences because of their drinking or illicit drug use. Most commonly these related to financial, domestic or legal problems. In addition 26 per cent of females and 22 per cent of males with such problems reported adverse consequences associated with their health. Smaller proportions also reported having encountered social or work-related difficulties.

The male and female prostitutes in this Edinburgh study were far from homogeneous. Some regarded themselves as full-time professionals, some of whom clearly disdained those who worked 'on the beat' (on the streets) or who used drugs intravenously. In spite of this, many of those who were included in this study had worked as prostitutes in a number of different settings. Some of those who currently worked in saunas and massage parlours had earlier worked for escort agencies, in bars or on the streets and there was clearly some movement between these different modes of operation. Overall, the results of this study, like the evidence reviewed in the previous section, failed to support the conclusion that alcohol consumption or illicit drug use *per se* did foster 'unsafe sex'. It was apparent that high-risk sex was influenced by a considerable number of factors. In Edinburgh in particular, and in much of Scotland, it appears that very few prostitutes have 'pimps'. The latter are important in some other areas and have been noted to be an important source of sexually transmitted diseases for the prostitutes with whom they have contact and over whom they exert control (Morgan Thomas 1995). Nevertheless, this study showed that many prostitutes report being asked by clients to engage in sex without condoms and that some did consent to this for extra payments. Moreover, most of the Edinburgh prostitutes reported having had recent sexual contact with lovers or other non-paying partners. Most of those who had regular non-paying partners rarely, if ever, used condoms with these individuals. Approximately 60 per cent of the men and women in this study reported having had an HIV test, though not necessarily a recent one. Twelve females and five males reported that they were HIV infected. All of these males had used drugs intravenously and had shared injecting equipment. Nine of the females also had such a background.

> The remaining three females attributed their HIV infection to sexual transmission. One reported that her regular partner was a seropositive intravenous drug user. The other two reported that their former partners included people whom they knew were HIV seropositive. Both women also reported having had hepatitis B at least once. It is therefore probable that their sero-conversions were also related to intravenous drug use by their partners.
>
> (Morgan Thomas 1990: 101)

It is clear that levels of illicit drug use vary markedly amongst different groups of men and women who work in the sex industry. This has been emphasized by De Graaf *et al.* (1994), commenting on their findings in the Netherlands. These authors concluded that street working male prostitutes were more likely to use 'hard' drugs (such as heroin) than those who worked at home. Moreover, it was concluded that street working prostitutes were also more likely to be heterosexual, to have no other job, to have more clients, but fewer 'steady' ones and to have a 'more negative working attitude'. De Graaf and his colleagues noted that homosexual prostitution brings together gay men and injecting drug users. They further commented that both of these sub-groups have high rates of HIV infection. This Dutch study indicated that most of the male prostitutes who were intravenous drug users had been drug dependent before beginning to work in the sex industry:

> While they did use their earnings from prostitution to pay for their addiction, only very few ever felt compelled to recruit customers while 'sick', i.e. in acute need of drugs. When that did happen, they were seldom particular about their choice of client.
>
> (De Graaf *et al.* 1994: 279)

De Graaf *et al.* also commented that of the men they interviewed who consumed alcohol while contacting clients: 'Alcohol use was highest among those who recruited clients in bars: they took, on average, 12 glasses when they worked, compared to eight glasses for the whole group of alcohol drinkers'. (1994: 279). De Graaf *et al.* concluded that men already using 'hard drugs' became prostitutes in order to finance their drug dependence and as an alternative to crime. They also noted: 'drug users were caught in a vicious circle out of which they knew no way' (1994: 281).

Another Dutch report concluded that drinking and illicit drug use by heterosexual and homosexual prostitutes was common (De Graaf *et al.* 1995). The authors noted that consumption patterns varied amongst different subgroups of people:

> Those meeting their clients in clubs or bars reported the highest consumption of alcohol; hard drugs were used predominantly by street prostitutes. It appears that the main effects of alcohol and drug use are on how the individual experiences working as, or calling on, a prostitute, the social interaction between the two parties and the sexual contact itself. The common assumption that drinking has negative effects on condom use was not borne out; though female prostitutes under the influence of drugs were significantly more likely to report unsafe sex.
>
> (De Graaf *et al.* 1995: 35)

Studies from Glasgow, only 60 kilometres west of Edinburgh, have shown a very different pattern from that evident in the Scottish capital (McKeganey and Barnard 1992). It has been reported that street prostitution, often involving intravenous drug users, is extremely widespread in Glasgow. For example, McKeganey *et al.* (1990) reported that roughly 300 women worked as street prostitutes in Glasgow's red-light area and that 60 per cent of those were intravenous drug users. McKeganey *et al.* (1992) further reported that of a study group of 206 street working females, 71 per cent were injecting drug users. Of those in this investigation who were HIV tested, 2.5 per cent were found to be HIV infected. Taylor *et al.* (1993) have described fifty-one female drug-injecting prostitutes in Glasgow. These authors reported that 45 per cent of these women had injected with used needles and syringes in the previous month. It was also noted that condom use with clients was 'almost universal', but was low with non-paying partners. Another Glasgow study examined HIV prevalence amongst female street prostitutes attending a health care drop-in centre. This indicated that 4.7 per cent of the intravenous drug users tested were HIV infected (Carr *et al.* 1992). All infected individuals were intravenous injectors. Another Glasgow study elicited HIV test information from female prostitutes who were intravenous drug users. Different methods were used to study subjects. HIV prevalence rates ranged from 1.2 per cent to 4.7 per cent (Goldberg *et al.* 1994). Green *et al.* (1993: 1581) have reported that some female prostitutes attending a Glasgow drop-in centre were engaging in a practice known as 'frontloading':

> Frontloading is used by two or more injectors to share out drugs. The injector draws up the drug solution from a preparatory vessel ('cooker') into his/her own syringe and then injects ('spouts') a proportion of the solution directly into the barrel of his/her colleague's syringe.

Gossop *et al.* (1993) have reported that, amongst London heroin users, the severity of drug dependence was positively associated with the frequency with which they had engaged in sex for either money or drugs. These authors commented that this connection applied to females as well as to men who had sex with men. Generally low levels of condom use were higher in contacts involving payment than in those with non-paying partners. This disparity has also been reported by other commentators (e.g. Morgan Thomas 1990; Morgan Thomas *et al.* 1990b; Taylor *et al.* 1993). The fact that prostitutes are less likely to use condoms with lovers than with paying clients is not surprising. For many people, using a condom is not only a public health measure. It is a barrier to intimacy and trust. Rhodes *et al.* (1994) examined female drug injectors in London, some of whom were engaged in prostitution. The latter were significantly more likely to be in contact with drug treatment agencies and to have had an HIV test than were the non-prostitutes. There were no significant differences between prostitutes and non-prostitutes in levels of HIV infection (12.9 per cent and 14.2 per cent respectively). These findings lend support to the conclusion that the major HIV risk for British prostitutes appear to come from intravenous drug use, rather than through prostitution in itself.

Gossop *et al.* (1994) have also stated that there were high levels of alcohol intoxication amongst prostitutes in south London. Matthews (1990) had commented upon high levels of alcohol and illicit drug use amongst female street working prostitutes in Liverpool. Morrison *et al.* (1994) reported that 10.5 per cent of a study group of female prostitutes in Liverpool had consumed more than 30 units of alcohol per week. This group had a mean week's consumption of over 200 units. The majority of Liverpool prostitutes surveyed, 67 per cent, reported working under the influence of alcohol. Half had used drugs intravenously.

The possible role of alcohol and illicit drugs has been discussed by Morrison *et al.* (1995). These commentators noted:

> The most inebriated prostitutes on the street appear to be the most successful in attracting clients. Women who appear entirely powerless and incapable of setting the boundaries of sexual activity to take place will attract men who may wish to legitimate an act of sexual abuse by the payment of cash.
>
> We feel that a distinction must be made between escort prostitution and street prostitution. A contract between a sex trade client and an escort prostitute may be one of equal partners and she will have the choice to decline business unacceptable to her. In street prostitutes, who are funding their dependence on alcohol or drugs, the power is with clients who have the money to set the agenda for the type of sex they want.
>
> (1995: 292)

Drug use by prostitutes has periodically been noted as having clear health risks. Bloor *et al.* (1991) have speculated that an increase in Temazepam use by prostitutes might reduce levels of condom use with their clients. Syphilis has been associated with drug use amongst female prostitutes in Connecticut and amongst both male and female prostitutes in Amsterdam (Farley *et al.* 1990; van den Hoek *et al.* 1990). Intravenous drug use has been found to be associated with HIV infection amongst male prostitutes in the USA. This study also found that the use of 'crack' in the past month had been reported by 54.9 per cent of those studied, while 35 per cent had histories of intravenous drug use (Elifson *et al.* 1993). Another US study supported the conclusion that crack smokers in three cities were more likely than non-smokers to engage in both prostitution and high-risk sex (Edlin *et al.* 1992). A Dutch study of male drug users supported the conclusion that duration of intravenous drug use was positively associated with HIV infection. A fifth of the men in this study had worked as prostitutes (van den Hoek *et al.* 1991).

An Australian study of female prostitutes and other women at the Sydney STD centre indicated that cannabis was the most widely used illicit drug by both groups. Other substances used were sleeping pills, amphetamines, cocaine and heroin. The prostitutes were more likely than the other women to smoke tobacco. In contrast, however, the prostitutes were less likely to drink, but were more likely to do so at a harmful level if they did consume alcohol (Philpot *et al.* 1989).

SEX INDUSTRY CLIENTS

As part of the Edinburgh study noted above, information was obtained about alcohol and drug use by clients, those who purchased sexual services. These details were elicited in two ways. First, the male and female prostitutes who were interviewed were asked to comment upon the proportions of their own clients who, in their view, appeared to be under the influence of alcohol or illicit drugs at the time of contact. These individuals indicated that approximately two-thirds of their clients appeared or were believed to have been drinking and that roughly a third appeared to have been using illicit drugs such as cannabis. It is emphasized that such reports were purely subjective. They did not necessarily imply intoxication nor even heavy alcohol/drug use by clients, simply perceived or apparent use (M.L. Plant *et al.* 1990). The second approach to clients involved direct interviews with a non-randomly contacted study group of 206 males and three females who had obtained sex in exchange for some form of payment (Morgan Thomas *et al.* 1990a). Most of the clients interviewed were men who had contacted prostitutes through saunas and massage parlours. Twenty-six of these men had contacted male prostitutes, five had contacted both males and females. One of the female clients had paid for sex with both men and women. Two had paid for sex with males.

Twenty-six of the male clients reported having at some time used drugs intravenously, of whom twenty-two also stated that they had at some time shared injecting equipment. Seven men reported that they were HIV infected. All of these had histories of intravenous drug use. Most of the men interviewed, 78 per cent, reported that drinking was sometimes a feature of their contacts with prostitutes. In addition 12 per cent stated that they 'usually' or 'always' used illicit drugs while in contact with prostitutes.

A further 17 per cent indicated that they 'sometimes' used drugs while in contact with prostitutes.

Only ten clients reported being non-drinkers. The mean alcohol consumption of the male clients who did drink was 10.6 units of alcohol. Twenty-five men (12 per cent) had consumed more than 50 units of alcohol in the past week. Consistent with the relatively heavy drinking of these clients, 71 per cent also smoked tobacco and 71 per cent also reported that they had smoked cannabis. Following a parallel procedure to that used in the survey of Edinburgh prostitutes (M.L. Plant *et al.* 1990), respondents were asked to assess the proportion of prostitutes with whom they had been in contact who were 'under the influence' of alcohol or illicit drugs at the time. The responses thus produced indicated that 69 per cent of male prostitutes and 38 per cent of females were judged to have been under the effects of alcohol. The corresponding proportions for perceived illicit drug effects were 40 per cent and 32 per cent. It should be noted that clients came from all socio-economic strata. These ranged from affluent and senior professionals to the unskilled, low paid or unemployed. No escort agency clients were, however, included in this study group. These clients, largely due to the way in which field-work was organized, were heavily skewed to emphasize men who visited massage parlours and saunas. Even so, a considerable proportion of those interviewed had contacted prostitutes in other ways, such as in hotels, bars, brothels, escort agencies or on the streets.

Consistent with the results of this Edinburgh study, De Graaf *et al.* (1995), commenting on the situation in the Netherlands, concluded that alcohol use by sex industry clients was common, though less so than amongst the prostitutes with whom they had contact.

CONCLUSIONS AND DISCUSSION

Not surprisingly, the evidence reviewed in this chapter supports the conclusion that the vast number of men and women in the sex industry do not conform to a single stereotype. These individuals come from a wide range of social backgrounds and work in a variety of different settings. Even so, it is also clear that the sex industry does sometimes attract alcohol- and drug-dependent people and that a high proportion of those in the sex industry are heavy users of alcohol, tobacco and illicit drugs. This certainly reflects many different factors: first, in some localities men and women work as prostitutes, most probably as street prostitutes, in order to pay for alcohol or drug supplies. Second, the working conditions and social milieu surrounding prostitution commonly foster the use of both licit and illicit psychoactive drugs. This reflects the fact that many prostitute–client contacts are made in and around bars, clubs and other licensed premises. It also probably reflects the fact that there is a strong occupational ethos of regular and heavy drinking, smoking and illicit drug use. Such a tradition is evident in a number of occupational groups (Plant 1979; Gill 1994; Hutcheson *et al.* 1995).

On the basis of the evidence reviewed above, it can reasonably be concluded that many of the prostitutes studied were heavy drinkers, and used both tobacco and illicit drugs, especially cannabis. A high proportion of street working prostitutes are clearly opiate users, intravenous drug users and drug dependants. Such findings are certainly distorted by the difficulty of obtaining a 'representative' sample of those engaged in an occupation that is, in most contexts, socially stigmatized and which often operates with some degree of secrecy.

In spite of the obvious methodological problems of conducting research into the sex industry, there is persuasive evidence to confirm the view that several areas of the sex industry do actively attract heavy drinkers or drug users, or foster such behaviour. Most, but not all, prostitutes are young. Most, but not all, come from working-class families. Many of those engaged in prostitution have little formal education and many are unmarried or without long-term partnerships. These demographic characteristics – youth, being unmarried and from working-class backgrounds – by themselves are consistent with relatively high levels of tobacco smoking and illicit drug use. The working environments of many of those in the sex industry also promote the social and convivial use of both legal and illicit drugs. Some of the individuals in the sex industry are professional prostitutes who work indoors in 'saunas', 'massage parlours' or brothels. Others work for escort agencies and often visit expensive hotels. Such individuals are clearly often very different from intravenous drug users who may engage in prostitution on a temporary basis to pay for their drug supplies. Heavy or problematic drinking or drug use are incompatible with some forms of sex work, such as for escort agencies and a number of indoor establishments. The managements of some agencies actively attempt to screen out and exclude individuals who are intravenous drug users or whose alcohol or drug use impedes work performance.

The use of alcohol, tobacco and illicit drugs is widespread amongst post-adolescents in most cultures. Sex, drinking, smoking, drug use and leisure are connected for a host of psychological and social reasons. The sex industry is not unique in its ability to bring these behaviours together. Most people use some form of psychoactive drug. What is striking about those engaged in the sex industry, either as prostitutes or as clients, is their variety, rather than their uniformity.

Afterword

Rethinking prostitution

Graham Scambler and Annette Scambler

INTRODUCTION

One of the principal motivations for this volume was to occasion and assist a rethinking of the institution of prostitution in Britain. It is apparent from recent discussions in the public sphere – involving not only academics, intellectuals and sex workers themselves, but politicians, the police, social and health workers and bodies like the Mothers' Union – that there is profound and widespread unease at the existing state of affairs. This is perhaps most obvious in relation to the law. It is clear that the anti-prostitution laws of the 1950s penalized women sex workers, especially street workers, while either proving ineffective against or ignoring other key participants in the sex industry, such as pimps, exploitative landlord and clients. Moreover, this legislation has now been exposed as unacceptably sexist. It was gender-biased even in conception: there was a High Court ruling on 5 May 1994, for example, that *only women* can be charged with loitering under the Street Offences Act of 1959.

As Shrage (1994: 82) notes, feminists who disagree markedly on the morality and symbolism of prostitution nevertheless tend to agree that 'the legal and political instruments available to control prostitution are problematic. In general, feminists who entertain the hope of eliminating sex commerce, and those who do not, all favour removing existing legal prohibitions against it.'

The fact of unease in the face of current legislation need not, then, imply a consensus around a programme of change. Debates about the rights and wrongs of prostitution, and what form of regulation – if any – it warrants, go back centuries (Roberts 1992). It is not possible to do justice to these debates here; but we want to close the volume by briefly addressing some of the social and moral issues raised by current dissensus and dispute. It will be expedient to consider first, selected *philosophical* reflections on these issues; second, to precis some *feminist* critiques; and finally, to comment on certain *pragmatic* considerations of policy and practice in Britain.

PHILOSOPHICAL REFLECTIONS

There have been several attempts recently to marshal philosophical arguments either for or against sex work. A paper by Ericsson (1980), which outlines and challenges the major arguments against sex work, has proved a particularly potent catalyst, eliciting a number of uncompromising responses. Ericsson points out that almost all extant philosophical treatments of prostitution seem to take it for granted that prostitution is undesirable, and he goes on to identify seven common 'charges' made against it. The first is that sex work is *intrinsically immoral*. Having considered possible historical and social antecedents for this conviction, Ericsson (1980: 338) offers a personal response: 'If two adults voluntarily consent to an economic arrangement concerning sexual activity and this activity takes place in private, it seem plainly absurd to maintain that there is something intrinsically wrong with it.' Moreover, any claim that prostitution is 'intrinsically wrong' would seem to rule out any possibility of rational discussion.

The second charge, which Ericsson (1980: 339) describes as *sentimentalist*, is that sex between prostitute and client is 'impoverished, cold and impersonal'. Ericsson's retort is that much sex, including intramarital sex, can share these same characteristics (i.e. is far from the sentimentalist's putative ideal); and he adds that sex without love is not necessarily 'bad' sex. He stresses too that the sex worker does not sell her body or vagina, but rather sexual *services*.

The third or *paternalist* charge is that sex workers are so vulnerable to assault and prone to physical and mental disorders associated with their work that steps should be taken to discourage recruitment to the industry and to aid rehabilitation thereafter. They are, in short, acting against their own interests. Ericsson (1980: 344) remarks that other occupations are no less hazardous, and that most of the problems experienced by sex workers are a function of 'the social anathema attached to their way of life'. We might, he suggests, take steps to minimize the risks of sex work rather than try to rehabilitate those who run them. And in what sense can voluntary adult sex workers be said to be acting against interests pre-defined for them by others?

The fourth charge, labelled *Marxist*, eschews moralism and instead sees the sex worker as the most degraded and miserable representative of an exploited class. Ericsson's rejoinder is that this analysis, purely derivative of Marx's critique of capitalism, is too general: not only has the institution of prostitution existed in primitive and feudal as well as capitalist societies, but, since it is not exclusively the product of 'economic factors', a transition to socialism would prove no panacea.

The fifth or *feminist* charge can, as we have intimated, take a multiplicity of forms. Crucial, however, is the contention that 'the relation between hooker and "John" is one of object to subject – the prostitute being reified into a mere object, a thing for the male's pleasure, lust and contempt . . . a piece of merchandise'. Moreover, prostitution is an unequal institution: 'it represents a way out of *misère sexuel* only for men' (Ericsson 1980: 348–9). Having noted in passing the existence of substantial numbers of male prostitutes in most modern urban centres, Ericsson reiterates his view that sex workers sell not themselves but sexual services. He (1980: 353) continues:

> Since when does the fact that we, when visiting a professional, are not interested in him or her as a person, but only in his or her professional performance, constitute a ground for saying that the professional is dehumanized, turned into an object?

And if the sex worker is treated as a means to an end, is the client any less so? We might, Ericsson (1980: 355) suggests, look upon sex and sexuality with:

> the same naturalness as upon our cravings for food and drink. And, contrary to popular belief, we may have something to learn from prostitution in this respect, namely, that coition resembles nourishment in that if it can not be obtained in any other way it can always be bought. And bought meals are not always the worst.

Commercialization is the sixth charge. At the core of this charge is the contention that prostitution encourages the growing commercialization of lifestyle. Ericsson's (1980: 356) counter is that the sex industry is in this respect a symptom not a cause: 'Capitalism is perfectly able to create commercialistic dystopias on its own. It hardly needs the aid of prostitution in the process.'

The final charge considered is that of a *disturbed emotional life*. Ericsson admits that some sex workers might well meet with emotional problems due to their work, but he insists that the prime source of such problems is the stigma and public antagonism heaped upon the industry. The salient concept here is that of 'secondary deviation' (Lemert 1967).

Some of the stronger rejoinders to Ericsson have come from feminists, whose arguments we shall sample next; but before we do so it should be recorded that while Ericsson (like some others – see Primoratz 1993) is at pains to dispute the rarely contested claim that 'prostitution is undesirable', he is *not* concerned to defend the counter-claim that 'prostitution is desirable'.

FEMINIST CRITIQUES

Shrage (1989: 37) succinctly capture the feminist quandry over sex work:

> Prostitution raises difficult issues for feminists. On the one hand, many feminists want to abolish discriminatory criminal statutes that are mostly used to harass and penalize prostitutes, and rarely to punish johns and pimps – laws which, for the most part, render prostitutes more vulnerable to exploitation by their male associates. On the other hand, most feminists find the prostitute's work morally and politically objectionable. In their view, women who provide sexual services for a fee submit to sexual domination by men, and suffer degradation by being treated as sexual commodities.

Perhaps it is not unreasonable to characterize the standpoint of a number of feminists by the slogan '*Against* prostitution. *For* prostitutes' (although the subtlety of this position has undoubtedly been lost on many sex workers: it is difficult for them to see as allies those apparently campaigning to render them redundant) (Scambler *et al.* 1990).

Shrage's (1989: 348) own strategy is to show that the sex industry, like others of our social institutions, is 'structured by deeply ingrained attitudes and values which are oppressive to women'. While Ericsson at least seems aware of this type of feminist claim, Pateman (1983) insists that what she terms his 'liberal contractarianism' necessarily denies him any effective means of rebuttal. Her stance differs from his in several important respects. For example, she maintains that prostitution is not simply the selling of sexual services; rather, 'when sex becomes a commodity in the capitalist market so, necessarily, do bodies and selves. . . . In prostitution, because of the relation between the commodity being marketed and the body, it is the body that is up for sale' (1983: 562).

She also disagrees with Ericsson's notion that sex work is like 'sex without love or mutual affection', arguing that

> the difference between sex without love and prostitution is not the difference between cooking at home and buying food in restaurants; the difference is that between the reciprocal expression of desire and unilateral subjection to sexual acts with the consolation of payment: it is the difference for women between freedom and subjection.
>
> (1983: 563)

Pateman (1983: 563) argues that Ericsson 'stands firmly in the patriarchal tradition' in that he discusses prostitution 'as a problem about the women who are prostitutes, and our attitudes to them, not a problem about the men who demand to buy them'. She rejects the view that prostitution is an example of a free contract between equal individuals in the market, insisting that for feminists it is not possible to separate sex from power. Indeed, 'prostitution is the public recognition of men as sexual masters; it puts submission on sale as a commodity in the market' (Pateman 1983: 564). Ericsson is in error, according to Pateman, in assuming that the (sexual) selves of women and men are interchangeable. 'This may appear radical', Pateman (1983: 565) remarks, 'but it is a purely abstract radicalism that reduces differentiated, gendered individuality to the seemingly natural, undifferentiated, and universal figure of the "individual" – which is an implicit generalizatisn of the masculine self.'

PRAGMATIC CONSIDERATIONS

Alongside philosophical reflections on and feminist critiques of the sex industry are more pragmatic concerns about what should be done. And such concerns have of necessity to be tailored to the possibilities afforded for change in contemporary – patriarchal and capitalist – Britain. It does not in our view follow that too many punches should be pulled. In discussing how best to meet the health needs of sex workers, we have elsewhere distinguished between three 'levels' of change: *operational*, *political* and *structural* (Scambler and Scambler 1994, 1995).

We used the term *operational* change to refer to formal health promotion or service initiatives overseen by health workers and allied experts which neither challenge nor threaten core social institutions. *Political* change refers to initiatives which bear on health but are beyond the conventional spheres of influence and authority of health workers to accomplish. Such change, typically requiring government action, increases awareness of core social institutions and may indirectly pose a challenge or threat to them. *Structural* change refers to fundamental revisions within core social institutions which have a bearing on health but are beyond the capacities of both health workers and government to deliver. Structural change typically requires a mobilization of mass public support which, in turn, typically requires sustained and organized extra-parliamentary political action.

We used these distinctions to argue that operational change, from outreach health promotion programmes to more user-friendly clinics, necessarily adds up to little more than an exercise in damage limitation; and that this is a function of the social marginalization of women sex workers in communities and the law, and their resultant suspicion of all branches of 'officialdom'. We went on to advocate political change, on health and other grounds, in the form of a decriminalization of the sex industry, which would both remove the anomaly of a gender-biased body of legislation exclusive to a particular area of work and prepare the ground for de-marginalizing women sex workers and restoring basic citizenship and other rights to them. Finally, we noted that the elimination of one set of gender-biased laws would leave much else intact, and made a case for structural change to address the systematic disadvantages facing women, and especially lone mothers, in the British labour and housing markets, maintaining that relative poverty and limited opportunity are necessary elements of any sociology of the sex industry.

Axiomatically, these distinctions have applicability beyond issues of health, and the case for further consideration of the potential for political and structural change pertinent to the British sex industry towards the close of the twentieth century seems unanswerable. Arguments around political change tend to focus on the law. While there is a consensus that the current law is untenable, opinions on appropriate reform are much more fragmented, and not only among philosophers and feminists. There has been some experimentation with 'tolerance zones', or designated areas where sex workers can work set hours under conditions laid down by local authorities (e.g. in Birmingham and Nottingham); but the two modes of reform most often discussed are *legalization* and *decriminalization.*

Legalization is generally accompanied by a system of registration for women sex workers, who have also to submit to 'rules' designed to protect public health and decency. This usually means that women are required to have regular health checks to retain their licences to work in specified houses or localities.

Legalization has attracted some support recently and there is evidence of public receptiveness (Carroll and Scambler 1992). In a much-publicized report in 1992 the Mothers' Union watered down its opposition to the legalization of brothels. Publics, if not necessarily clients, tend to be more tolerant of forms of sex work which are perceived to be clean, safe and invisible. However, many sex workers, including the International Committee for Prostitutes' Rights (ICPR) and the English Collective of Prostitutes (ECP), argue that legalization merely represents an alternative, and in some ways more blatant, male mode of control of female sexuality than exists under present statutes. Moreover in countries where legalization has been introduced (e.g. Germany) it has on the whole not proved 'successful', since many women are unwilling to provide assembly-line sex for taxed pay in a state brothel and prefer to work illegally. Some women barred from working legally because of sexually transmitted diseases or other sickness also continue outside the law. Most women working illegally are vulnerable, at risk of exploitation and abuse and beyond the reach and influence of health workers and other agencies.

Decriminalization, or the total abolition of laws and sentences which discriminate against women sex workers, has been the subject of sex worker campaigns in Britain – notably by the ECP – and elsewhere since the mid-1980s. The ICPR has supplemented its (global) call for the decriminalization of 'voluntary adult sex work' with demands also for appropriate regulation of third parties; the impartial enforcement of extant legislation against fraud, coercion, rape, child abuse and so on; the granting of human and civil rights for sex workers; the extension of the taxation and benefits system to sex workers; and help and support for women electing to leave the sex industry. These are among the key demands articulated in the ICPR's 'World Charter' (Pheterson 1989).

The decriminalization of adult sex work freely entered into would not put sex workers beyond the law; but it would eliminate the anomaly of an essentially sexist body of law exclusive to a particular area of work. Nor would decriminalization in this country solve the growing global problem of 'stolen lives' due to 'sexual trafficking' (Altink 1995; Edwards, this volume); but it would perhaps help loosen the grip of more or less organized crime syndicates and other criminals. It should be noted, however. that Matthews (1986) has taken a contrary view, namely, that decriminalization would in all likelihood *increase* the level of exploitation of prostitutes. Citing Wilson's (1983: 224) statement that 'wholesale de-criminalization would simply mean a free for all for men', he (1986: 199) suggests 'the removal of legal constraints would give a free hand to entrepreneurs to organize prostitution as a legitimate business. The criminalizing of prostitution by reducing its legitimacy also reduces the potential profit and thus the overall rate of exploitation.'

In preference to either legalization or de-criminalization, Matthews (1986: 204) advocates a 'radical regulationism'. This involves: (a) a clear commitment to general deterrence; (b) the reduction of annoyance, harassment and disturbance; (c) protection from coercion and exploitation; and (d) the reduction of the commercialization of prostitution. Shrage (1994) is sympathetic to Matthews' fourfold strategy, although she notes his lack of comment on the means for its effective implementation. She (1994: 159) expounds her own version as follows:

> It would be a system where prostitutes would not be 'registered' and brothels would not be 'licensed', but where prostitutes themselves would be licensed, much like other professionals and semi-professional. Since in the sex industry the primary productive assets are the bodies of sex providers, and the primary trade secrets are contained in their personal skills, knowledge, charm and talent, sex providers should be given as much control as possible over the operation and use of these talents.

The standards for licensing should be established by 'public boards or commissions made up of service providers, community leaders, educators and legal and public health experts'.

Shrage sees a number of advantages in licensing individual sex workers: it would allow sex workers to work for themselves or form cooperatives, which would leave them less vulnerable to large commercial interests; by controlling how their services were offered, it would render them less vulnerable too to clients, small-scale entrepreneurs, pimps and public officials; it would afford them semi-professional status, which would give them the authority to 'lead certain kinds of business and sexual transactions'; by engaging in sex work profitably, they might challenge the cultural association between sex and harm to women; by involving sex workers in designing and monitoring the procedures for licensing, it would empower those likely to protect sex workers' legal rights; and, finally, it would both give clients reassurance that certain standards would be met and 'provide the public with a vehicle for addressing possible hazards that might result from the industry'.

Legalization, decriminalization and regulationism have been introduced here as exemplars of political change and as ideal types; other – and 'mixed' – reform packages are possible. Our concern has been to trigger further debate in the public sphere on what almost all commentators agree is an unacceptable set of prostitution laws presently in force (in England and Wales). We have only been able in the confines of this Afterword to give a flavour of the pros and cons of select recipes for reform.

It is perhaps fitting to close with another reference to structural change. British women's continuing economic and hierarchic heterosexual dependencies are part and parcel of a comprehensive system of patriarchal institutions, norms and relationships, as are the constrained, marginal and often hazardous and health-exacting lives of contemporary women sex workers. Structural change towards the elimination of gender disadvantages in material and ideological circumstance, is in our view a precondition for the effectiveness of legal reform and for the reconstruction or 'displacement' of the flawed British sex industry of the 1990s via the empowerment through full citizenship of all its current sex workers.

Notes

1 PROSTITUTE WOMEN NOW

1 Glendenning states that Conservative economic and employment policies have hit women in paid work in three ways: women are increasingly vulnerable to redundancy and unemployment: restructuring the labour market adversely affects the types of jobs and pay women receive; and women's statutory rights are eroded when in work. Between 1979 and 1986 male unemployment rose by 143 per cent, female unemployment rose by 189 per cent (1987: 50–1).

2 From conversations with women working as prostitutes and women no longer working as prostitutes in Britain and Europe.

3 These points evolved out of discussions between members of the 'Prostitution and Feminism' workshop at the 1st European Whores Congress in Frankfurt am Main, October 1991. The workshop was led by Andre Gunter and Christiane Tillner.

4 From conversations with women working as prostitutes in the East Midlands and the Netherlands.

5 Rosemary Barbaret of the University of Seville and I are working on a collaborative study comparing the social organization of prostitution in Spain and England (urban and rural dimensions). The intention is to explore and develop policy-oriented recommendations. APRAMP are key players in the study of prostitution within the city of Madrid. We hope that the organization POW! in Nottingham and APRAMP can exchange skills and ideas for future practice.

6 POW! evolved out of a one-year research project conducted at the Department of Epidemiology and Public Health, Nottingham University. Women involved in researching (via snowballing techniques) the relationship between prostitution, drugs and HIV developed their own voluntary agency based upon principles of peer education with the support of staff at Nottingham University, Nottingham Trent University, the Probation Service, individuals working as researchers, a solicitor, health professionals, and members of the Church and the East Midlands Forum on Prostitution. Currently seeking charitable status POW! workers have developed the organization to address issues relating to: health, welfare and legal needs, drug related needs,

vocational guidance, education, training and counselling, the need for places of safety, and work with young people often under age and from local authority care. The philosophy of the organization is based upon principles of peer-led education and empowerment.

WHIP was started by volunteers from the following agencies, Leicestershire AIDS support services (LASS), and Drug Advice and Lesbian and Gay Line, and was launched in 1990. It was founded on the need to respond to problems experienced by working women around HIV prevention, education support, violence and welfare needs in collaboration with women working as prostitutes. There is one co-ordinator and ten volunteers. Women are contacted on an outreach basis on the street, in saunas and massage parlours, and via contact magazines. The project hopes to establish a drop-in centre where women can come for clinical, welfare and other advice. Further, the group are developing safe house facilities for women experiencing violence or escaping violent pimps, and who may want to leave prostitution and need a short-term refuge.

Soliciting for Change is coordinated by a youth worker who developed outreach work with female prostitutes on streets in the Caldmore area of Birmingham. With the backing of the local Church and professionals associated through the steering committee Soliciting for Change organized a local conference followed by a national conference to look at reforming the laws around prostitution. The national conference was held at Nottingham on 25–6 September 1993 and was a key-point in the development of a national platform for the human rights and civil liberties of women working as prostitutes.

SCOT-PEP are a peer-led education project founded in Edinburgh in the Spring of 1989. They are committed to 'harm reduction in relation to the sex industry and drug use. The project operates on a self-help model using the knowledge and expertise of prostitutes, drug users and others, with the intention of raising awareness of those still working and those entering the sex industry' Morgan Thomas (1993: 3). The aims are as follows:

- to enable prostitutes to minimise their risk of sexually transmitted diseases including HIV/Aids.
- to provide information and support around harm reduction in relation to HIV/Aids in the sex industry to male and female prostitutes, their partners and others involved
- to empower prostitutes, thereby enabling them to take full responsibility for their sexual health and maximise their quality of life within the sex industry
- to give prostitutes a voice in the HIV and Aids forum
- to work towards the harmonisation of legislation, law enforcement and public health interest.

(1993: 3)

2 PROSTITUTE MEN NOW

1 We use the term 'AIDS' to refer to the symbolic construction and social impact of HIV. The latter term we use to refer to the spectrum of physical manifestations of the virus.

2 That is to say there is no literature on the subject as far as we have been able to discover. Needless to say, literature is not the only way in which such ideas percolate and we may simply be unaware of groups and movements. Even if this is so, the main thrust of our argument is not affected.

3 Note that the figures in this section do not correspond directly with those in the last. This is because of a complicated data collection method which confused us, the interviewer and those interviewed. We are treating the two data sources as internally consistent, which seems reasonable, but not trying to cross-validate the data. However, the difference between the estimates in the recall of partners and the estimates in the *N* of acts, the average discrepancy is only 10 per cent, which gives some confidence in the validity of the data.

4 CAMPAIGNING FOR LEGAL CHANGE

1 On 27 August 1981 – after the 1980 and 1981 street rebellions led by young Black people in many British cities and a long opposition from Black and other civil rights organizations – the 'sus' law was repealed and replaced by the Criminal Attempts Act. Under the old law anyone could be arrested and charged by police on the grounds that being a 'suspected' person, s/he was loitering with intent to commit an arrestable offence. It was used to police youths, especially Black youths, in London and other big cities, who were on the street at times when they 'should' have been at work or in school. 'Sus' became an easy arrest for young police looking to earn their promotion. There were two standard versions: (1) the accused was seen looking into cars and trying the door handles, and (2) the accused was seen dipping his/her hands into women's handbags in bus queues. Only police evidence was necessary. There was never a case where the woman victim was called on as a witness. In nearly all cases magistrates rubber-stamped the police evidence, unless the accused was lucky enough to have something like a clocking-out card to prove he was at work at the time he was supposed to be at a particular bus-stop.

2 Lindi St Clair's 'Prostitution Dossier', House of Commons Library, November 1991.

3 ECP letter to Attorney General re Pat Malone. It was endorsed by over 80 organizations.

4 Office for AIDS Surveillance, New York, 31 October 1991, and San Francisco, 31 May 1992; *UK Parliamentary AIDS Digest*, Spring 1991.

5 ECP press release, 13 July 1992.

7 HEALTH CARE AND REGULATION

Thanks to the Medical Research Council, AVERT, North West Thames Regional Health Authority and the Jefferiss Trust for financial support, and to the founding members of the Praed Street Project team – Catrina Donegan, Louise Hanson, Jane Mezzone – and to all staff and users of the Praed Street Project.

1 Where case histories are presented, names and various details have been changed to preserve confidentiality.
2 The use of the services was not conditional on taking part in the research.

8 ALCOHOL, DRUGS AND SOCIAL MILIEU

The author is extremely grateful to Dr Moira Plant of the Alcohol Research Group and Ms Ruth Morgan Thomas of the Scottish Prostitutes' Education Project (SCOT-PEP), Edinburgh for some of the information presented in this chapter.

The Edinburgh study was supported by the Medical Research Council with additional support from the Scotch Whisky Association, the Bill Kenyon Education Trust, the Scottish Health Education Group, an anonymous charity and the Portman Group.

References

FOREWORD: UNDERSTANDING PROSTITUTION

Bassermann, L. (1967) *The Oldest Profession: A History of Prostitution*, London: Arthur Barker Ltd.

Beck, U. and Beck-Gernsheim, E. (1995) *The Normal Chaos of Love*, Cambridge: Polity Press.

Berger, P., Berger, B. and Kellner, H. (1973) *The Homeless Mind: Modernization and Consciousness*, New York: Allen Lane.

Brittan, A. (1989) *Masculinity and Power*, Oxford: Blackwell.

English Collective of Prostitutes (1992) *Prostitute Women and AIDS: Resisting the Virus of Repression*, London: Crossroads Books.

Giddens, A. (1990) *Consequences of Modernity*, Cambridge; Polity Press.

Giddens, A. (1992) *The Transformation of Intimacy: Sexuality, Love and Eroticism in Modern Society*, Cambridge: Polity Press.

Habermas, J. (1984) *Theory of Communicative Action, Vol. 1. Reason and the Rationalization of Society*, Cambridge: Polity Press.

Habermas, J. (1987) *Theory of Communicative Action, Vol. 2. Lifeworld and System*, Cambridge: Polity Press.

Lister, R. (1992) *Women's Economic Dependency and Social Security*, Manchester: Equal Opportunities Commission.

McLeod, E. (1982) *Working Women: Prostitution Now*, London: Croom Helm.

Merton, R. (1968) *Social Theory and Social Structure*, New York: Free Press.

Morris, L. (1994) *Dangerous Classes: The Underclass and Social Citizenship*, London: Routledge.

Muir, J. and Ross, M. (1993) *Housing the Poorer Sex*, London: London Housing Unit.

Oppenheim, C. (1990) *Poverty: The Facts*, London: Child Poverty Action Group.

Roberts, N. (1992) *Whores in History: Prostitution in Western Society*, London: HarperCollins.

Scambler, G. (1987) 'Habermas and the power of medical expertise', in G. Scambler (ed.) *Sociological Theory and Medical Sociology*, London: Tavistock.

Scambler, G., Peswani, R., Renton, A. and Scambler, A. (1990) 'Women prostitutes in the AIDS era', *Sociology of Health and Illness* 12: 260–73.

Shrage, L. (1989) 'Should feminists oppose prostitution?' *Ethics* 99: 347–61.

Truong, T.-D. (1990) *Sex, Money and Morality: Prostitution and Tourism in South-East Asia*, London: Zed Books.

1 PROSTITUTE WOMEN NOW

Barry, K. (1979) *Female Sexual Slavery*, New York: New York University Press.

Barry, K. (1988) 'Female sexual slavery: the problem, policies and cause for feminist action', in E. Boneparth and E. Stoper (eds) *Women, Power and Policy: towards the year 2000*, Oxford: Pergamon Press.

Barton, S. E., Taylor-Robinson, D. and Harris, J.R.W. (1987) 'Female prostitutes and sexually transmitted diseases', *British Journal of Hospital Medicine* 38.

Beck, U. (1992) *Risk Society: Towards a New Modernity*, London: Sage.

Benjamin, H. and Masters, R.E.L. (1965) *Prostitution and Morality*, London: Souvenir Press.

Bertilson, M. (1986) 'Love's labour lost? A sociological view', *Theory, Culture and Society* 3 (2) 19–35.

Biehal, N. *et al.* (1992) *Prepared for Living: A Survey of Young People Leaving the Care of Three Local Authorities*, Leeds University.

Boutellier, J. (1991) 'Prostitution, criminal law and morality in the Netherlands', *Crime, Law and Social Change* 15: 201–11.

Bullough, V. and Bullough, B. (1987) *Women and Prostitution: A Social History*, New York: Prometheus Books.

Company (1990) 'Executive by day, prostitute by night', *Company* Nov.: 42–3.

Connell, R.W. (1987) *Gender and Power*, Cambridge: Polity Press.

Corbin, A. (1987) 'Commercial sexuality in nineteenth-century France: a system of images and regulations', in C. Gallagher and T. Laquer (eds) *The Making of the Modern Body: Sexuality and Society in the Nineteenth Century*, Berkeley: University of California Press.

Corbin, A. (1990) *Women for Hire: Prostitution and Sexuality in France after 1850*, Cambridge, MA: Harvard University Press.

Day, S. (1990) 'Prostitute women and the ideology of work in London', in D.A. Feldman (ed.) *Culture and AIDS*, New York/London: Praeger.

Delacoste, F. and Alexander, P. (eds) (1988) *Sex Work: Writings by Women in the Sex Industry*, London: Virago.

Dibblin, J. (1991) *Wherever I Lay my Hat: Young Women and Homelessness*, London: Shelter.

Drobler, C. (1991) *Women at Work*, Reader 1st European Prostitutes' Congress, Frankfurt, October.

Edwards, S. (1988a) 'Policing street prostitution: the street offences squad in London', *Police Journal* July: 209–19.

Edwards, S. (1988b) *Prostitution, Policing. Employment and the Welfare of Young Women*, Report prepared for the Nuffield Foundation, Oxford.

Finnegan, F. (1979) *Poverty and Prostitution: A Study of Victorian Prostitutes in York*, Cambridge: Cambridge University Press.

Forum (1989) 'Interview with the Praed St Project', *Forum* 22(7): 33–41.

Fromm, E. (1967) *The Art of Loving*, London: Unwin.

Giddens, A. (1984) *The Constitution of Society*, Cambridge: Polity Press.

Giddens, A. (1992) *The Transformation of Intimacy: Sexuality, Love and Eroticism in Modern Societies*, Cambridge: Polity Press.

Glendinning, C. (1987) 'Impoverishing women', in A. Walker and C. Walker (eds) *The Growing Divide*, London: Child Poverty Action Group.

Golding, R. (1992) 'Policing prostitution', *Police Review* 8: 60–72.

Green, J. (1992) *Its No Game: Responding to the Needs of Young Women at Risk or Involved in Prostitution*, Leicester: National Youth Agency.

Grover, J.Z. (1989) 'AIDS: Keywords', in Crimp, D. (ed), *AIDS: Cultural Analysis, Cultural Activism*, Cambridge: MIT Press.

Hanmer, J. and Maynard, M. (eds) (1987) *Women, Violence and Social Control*, London: Macmillan.

Hanmer, J. and Saunders, S. (1984) *Well-founded Fear*, London: Hutchinson.

Hanmer, J., Radford, J. and Stanko, E. (1989) *Women. Policing and Male Violence*, London: Routledge.

Haraway, D. (1991) *Simians, Cyborgs and Women: The Reinvention of Nature*, London: Free Association Books.

Haug, F. (1992) *Beyond Female Masochism: Memory-works and Politics*, London: Verso.

Henriques, F. (1962) *Prostitution and Society: A Survey, Vol. 1: Primitive, Classical an Oriental*, London: MacGibbon & Kee.

Hoigard, C. and Finstad, L. (1992) *Backstreets Money, Prostitution and Love*, Cambridge: Polity Press.

Jackson, S. (1993) 'Even sociologists fall in love', *Sociology* 27 (2): 201–20.

Jaget, C. (ed.) (1980) *Prostitutes: Our Life*, Bristol: Falling Wall Press.

Jennes, V. (1990) 'From sex to sin to sex as work: COYOTE and the reorganization of Prostitution as a Social Problem', *Social Problems* 37 (3).

Jennes, V. (1993) *Making it Work: The Prostitutes' Rights Movement in Perspective*, New York: Aldine de Gruyter.

Kelly, L. (1988) *Surviving Sexual Violence*, Cambridge: Polity Press.

Kinnell, H. (1989) *Prostitutes, their Clients and Risks of HIV Infection in Birmingham*, Occasional Paper, Dept of Public Health Medicine, Birmingham.

Kinnell, H. (1991) *Safe: HIV Prevention Project*, collection of unpublished papers, Dept of Public Health and Medicine, Birmingham.

Kinsey, A. C. (1948) *Sexual Behaviour in the Human Male*, London: W.B. Saunders Co.

Kishtainy, K. (1982) *The Prostitute in Progressive Literature*, London: Allison & Busby.

Kruhse-Mountburton, S. (1992) 'An evaluation of Australian legislation on prostitution' in P. Van de Vort and P.M. Bruylant *La Prostitution,*

Quarante ans Après La Convention de New York, Ecole des Sciences Criminologiques Leon Cornil, Brussels.

Lees, S. (1993) *Sugar and Spice: Sexuality and Adolescent Girls*, London: Penguin.

Leukefeld, C.J., Battjes, R.J. and Amsel, Z. (eds) (1990) AIDS and Intravenous Drug Use: Community Intervention and Prevention, London: Hemisphere.

Lowman, J. (1992a) 'Correspondence', *British Journal of Criminology* 32 (3).

Lowman, J. (1992b) 'Street prostitution control: some Canadian reflections on the Finsbury Park experience', *British Journal of Criminology* 32 (1).

Luhmann, N. (1986) *Love as Passion*, Cambridge: Polity Press.

Lupton, C. (1985) *Moving Out*, Portsmouth Social Services Research Unit.

McIntosh, M. (1978) 'Who needs prostitutes? The ideology of male sexual needs', in C. Smart and B. Smart (eds) *Women, Sexuality and Social Control*, London: Routledge.

McKeganey, N. (1992) 'Hooked on the killing game', *Times Higher Educational Supplement* 3 July.

McKeganey, N. and Barnard, M. (1992a) *Aids, Drugs and Sexual Risk: Lives in the Balance*, Milton Keynes: Open University Press.

McKeganey, N. and Barnard, M. (1992b) 'Selling sex: female street prostitution and HIV risk behaviour in Glasgow', *AIDS* 4 (4): 395–407.

McKeganey, N., Barnard, M., Bloor, M. and Leyland, A. (1990) 'Injecting drug use and female street-working prostitution in Glasgow', *AIDS* 4: 1153–5.

McKeganey, N., Barnard, M., Leyland, A., Coote, I. and Follet, E. (1992) 'Female streetworking prostitution and HIV infection in Glasgow', *British Medical Journal* 305: 801–4.

McLeod, E. (1982) *Women Working: Prostitution Now*, London: Croom Helm.

McLintock, A. (1992) 'Gonad the Barbarian and the Venus FlyTrap: portraying the female and male orgasm', in L. Segal and M. McIntosh (eds) *Sex Exposed: Sexuality and the Pornography Debate*, London: Virago.

Matthews, R. (1986) 'Beyond Wolfenden? Prostitution, politics and the law', in R. Matthews and J. Young (eds) *Confronting Crime*, London: Sage.

Matthews, R. (1991) *Prostitution, Drugs and HIV: A Survey of Outreach Work with Young People*, Report for Sefton Youth Service.

Meil Hobson, B. (1990) *Uneasy Virtue: The Politics of Prostitution and the American Reform Tradition*, Chicago: University of Chicago Press.

Morgan-Thomas, R., Plant, M.A., Plant, M.L. and Sales, D.I. (1989) 'Risk of AIDS among workers in the "sex industry": some initial results from a Scottish study', *British Medical Journal* 299: 148–9.

Morgan, Thomas, R., Plant, M.A., Plant, M.L. and Sales, D.I. (1990) 'Risk of HIV infection among clients of the sex industry in Scotland', *British Medical Journal* 301: 525.

Newman, C. (1989) *Young Runaways: Findings from Britain's First Safe House*, London: Children's Society.

New Statesman and Society (1990) *'Tis no Pity she's a Whore*, 9 Feb.
O'Mahoney, B. (1988) *A Capital Offence: The Plight of the Young Single Homeless in London*, London: Routledge and Barnardos.
O'Neill, M. (1991) *Towards a Multi-agency Approach to Prostitution in Nottingham*, pilot study undertaken for 'Nottingham Safer Cities Project', Nottingham Polytechnic.
O'Neill, M. (1992) 'Women at Work: prostitution and feminism in the context of later modernity', *Phoebe* (interdisciplinary journal of feminist scholarship, theory and aesthetics) 4.
O'Neill, M. (1993a) *A Collection of Papers and Reports Documenting a 'Woman-centred' Multi-agency Approach to Prostitution*, Unpublished.
O'Neill, M. (1993b) 'Pimps and punters: the gendere organisation of female prostitution in conditions of later modernity', S. Stanko and J. Kimber (eds) *Masculinity and Crime: Issues of Theory and Practice*, Conference Report, Centre for Criminal Justice Research, Brunel, University of West London.
O'Neill, M. (1994) 'Prostitution and the state: towards a feminist practice' in C. Lupton and T. Gillespie (eds) *Working with Violence: Dilemmas for a Feminist Practice*, London: Macmillan.
O'Neill, M. (1995) 'Prostitution and violence: towards a feminist praxis', in J. Radford, M. Hester and L. Kelly (eds) *Women, Violence and Male Power: Feminist Activism, Research and Practice*, Oxford: Open University Press.
O'Neill, M., Goode, *et al.* (1995a) 'Juvenile prostitution – the experience of young women in residential care', *Childright* January.
O'Neill, M., Johnson, McDonald, Wellik, Webster, and McGregor, (1995b) *Prostitution, Feminism and the Law: Feminist Ways of Seeing, Knowing and Working with People Working with Prostitutes*, London: Rights of Women Bulletin.
Pateman, C. (1983) 'Defending prostitution: charges against Ericsson', *Ethics* April: 561–5.
Pheterson, G. (1986) *The Whore Stigma: Female Dishonor and Male Unworthiness*, Report Sponsored by the Dutch Ministry of Social Affairs and Employment, Emancipation Policy Coordination, the Netherlands.
Pheterson, G. (ed.) (1989) *A Vindication of the Rights of Whores*, Seattle: Seal Press.
Pheterson, G. (1990) 'The category "prostitute" in scientific enquiry', *Journal of Sex Research* 27 (3): 397–407.
Plant, M. (ed.) (1990) *AIDS, Drugs and Prostitution*, London: Routledge.
Pollak, M. (1988) *Les Homosexuels et le SIDA: Sociologie d'une Épidémie*, Paris: Métailié.
Radford, J. and Russell, D. (eds) (1992) *Femicide: The Politics of Women Killing*, Milton Keynes: Open University Press.
Roberts, N. (1992) *Whores in History*, London: HarperCollins.
Ryle, C. (1992) *Prostitution: Report for Community Affairs Division*, Birmingham City Council.
Scambler, G. and Scambler, A. (1992) 'Health issues for women prostitutes in London: a preliminary report', unpublished discussion paper.

Scambler, G., Peswani, R., Renton, A. and Scambler. A. (1990) 'Women prostitutes in the AIDS era', *Sociology of Health and Illness* 12 (3).
Shedlin, M. (1990) 'An Ethnographic Approach to Understanding HIV High-Risk Behaviours: Prostitution and Drug Abuse', in Leukefeld, C.G., Battjes, R.J. and Amsel, Z. (eds) *AIDS and intravenous drug use: community intervention and prevention*, USA Hemisphere Publishing Corporation.
Smart, C. (1992) *Regulating Womanhood: Historical Essays on Marriage, Motherhood and Sexuality*, London: Routledge.
Smith, D. (1993) *Texts, Facts, and Femininity: Exploring the Relations of Ruling*, London: Routledge.
Stanley, L. (ed.) (1990) *Feminist Praxis*, London: Routledge.
Stein, M. (1990) *Living out of Care*, London: Barnardos.
Stein, M. (1991) *Leaving Care and the 1989 Children Act*, First Key.
Sunday Correspondent (1990) 'Students on the game', 25 Nov.
Video Diaries (1993) BBC 2.
Walby, S. (1989) *Theorizing Patriarchy*, Cambridge: Polity Press.
Walklate, S. (1991) *Teenage Prostitution in Sefton*, Sefton Youth Service.
Walkowitz, J. (1980) *Prostitution in Victorian Society*, Cambridge: Cambridge University Press.
Welzer-Lang, D. (1993) 'Prostitution from tradition to modernity', interim report of work in progress, University of Lyon, France.
Wolfenden Committee (1957) *Report on Homosexuality and Prostitution*, CMND 24722, London: HMSO.
Zola, E. (1972) *Nana*, Harmondsworth: Penguin.

2 PROSTITUTE MEN NOW

Altman, D. (1986) *AIDS and the New Puritanism*, Pluto: London.
Barry, K. (1979) *Female Sexual Slavery*, New York: Avon.
Butts, W.M. (1947) 'Boy prostitutes of the metropolis', *Journal of Clinical Psychopathology* 8: 673–81.
Chiasson, M.A., Lifson, A.R., Stoneburner, R.L. and Ewing, W. *et al.* (1988) 'HIV seroprevalence in male and female prostitutes in New York City', paper presented at the IVth International Conference on AIDS, Stockholm.
Coombs, N.R. (1974) 'Male prostitution: a psychosocial view of behaviour', *American Journal of Orthopsychiatry* 55 (5): 782–9.
Coutinho, R.A., van Andel, R.L.M. and Rijsdijk, T.J. (1988) 'Role of male prostitutes in the spread of Sexually Transmitted Diseases and Human Immunodeficiency Virus', *Genitourinary Medicine* 64: 207–8.
Darrow, W. (1992) 'Assessing targeted AIDS prevention in male and female prostitutes and their clients', in Paccaud, F., Vader, J. P. and Gutzwiler (eds), *Assessing AIDS Prevention*, Basel: Birkhauser Verlag, p. 215.
Davies, P.M. and Project SIGMA (1992) 'On relapse: recidivism, or rational response?' in P. Aggleton, P.M. Davies and G. Hart (eds) *AIDS: Rights, risk and Reason*, London: Falmer.
Davies, P.M. and Simpson, P. (1990) 'On male homosexual prostitution and

HIV', in P. Aggleton, P.M. Davies and G. Hart (eds) *AIDS: Individual, Cultural and Policy Dimensions*, London: Falmer, pp. 103–20.

Davies, P.M. and Weatherburn P. (1991) 'Towards a general model of sexual negotiation', in P. Aggleton, P.M. Davies and G. Hart (eds) *AIDS: Response, Interventions and Care*, London: Falmer, pp. 111–26.

Davies, P.M., Hickson, F.C.I., Weatherburn, P. and Hunt, A.J. (1993) *Sex, Gay Men and AIDS*, London: Falmer Press.

Day, S. (1989) 'Prostitute women and the ideology of lover in London', paper presented at the 3rd Conference on the Social Aspects of AIDS, London.

Elifson, K.W., Boles, J., Sweat, M. and Darrow, W.W. *et al.* (1988) 'Seroprevalence of Human Immunodeficiency Virus among male prostitutes', *New England Journal of Medicine* 321: 832–3.

Harris, M. (1973) *The Dilly Boys*, London: Croom Helm.

Hickson, F.C.I., Weatherburn, P., Hows, J. and Davies, P.M. (1994) 'Selling Safer Sex: Male Masseurs and Escorts in the U.K.', in Aggleton, P., Davies, P.M. and Hart, G. (eds) *AIDS: Foundations for the Future*, London: Falmer, pp. 197–209.

Kinnell, H. (1991) 'Prostitutes' perceptions of risk and factors related to risk-taking', in P. Aggleton, P.M. Davies and G. Hart (eds) *AIDS: Responses, Interventions and Care*, London: Falmer Press, pp. 79–94.

Kooistra, O. and Hazenkamp, J.L. (1992) 'Streetwise: survival of boys in prostitution', paper presented at the 2nd Conference on Homosexuality and HIV, Amsterdam.

Lloyd, R. (1979) *Playland: A Study of Human Exploitation*, London: Quartet.

Marotta, T., Waldorf, D. and Murphy, S. (1988) 'Males doing sex-work in the San Francisco Bay area: a typology and description', unpublished paper, Institute for Scientific Analysis, San Francisco.

McMullen, R. (1988) 'Youth prostitution: a balance of power', *Journal of Adolescence* 10: 33–43.

Reiss, A.J. (1961) 'The social integration of queers and peers', *Social Problems* 9: 102–19.

Robinson, T.J. and Davies, P.M. (1991) 'London's homosexual male prostitutes: power, peer groups and HIV', in P. Aggleton, P.M. Davies and G. Hart (eds) *AIDS: Response, Interventions and Care*, London: Falmer, pp. 95–110.

Tirelli, U., Vaccher, E., Bullian, P. and Saracchini, S. *et al.* (1988) 'HIV-1 seroprevalence in male prostitutes in Northeast Italy', *Journal of Acquired Immunodeficiency Syndrome* I: 414–17.

van de Lagemaat, G. (1986) 'The making of the modern business boy', unpublished paper, University of Utrecht.

Watney, S. (1987) *Policing Desire: Pornography, AIDS and the Media*, Comedia: London.

Weatherburn, P. and Project SIGMA (1992) in P. Aggleton, P.M. Davies and G. Hart (eds) *AIDS: Rights, Risk and Reason*, London: Falmer Press.

Weeks, J. (1989) 'AIDS: the intellectual agenda', in P. Aggleton, P.M. Davies and G. Hart (eds) *AIDS: Social Representations, Social Practices*, London: Falmer Press, pp. 1–20.

West, D.J. with de Villiers, B. (1992) *Male Prostitution*, London: Duckworth.

3 THE LEGAL REGULATION OF PROSTITUTION

Barnard, M.A. (1993) 'Violence and vulnerability: conditions of work for streetwalking prostitutes', *Sociology of Health and Illness* 15 (5): 681–705.

Barry, K. (1981) *Female Sexual Slavery*, New York: New York University Press.

Chambers, G. and Millar, A. (1983) *Investigating Sexual Assault*, Scottish Home and Health Department: Edinburgh.

Chambers, G. and Millar, A. (1986) *Prosecuting Sexual Assault*, Scottish Home and Health Department: Edinburgh.

Coleman, F. and McMurtrie, S. (1993) 'Too hot to handle', *New Law Journal* 143 (8 Jan): 10–11.

Criminal Statistics, Supplementary Tables 1990, 1991, 1992, 1993, London: Government Statistical Office.

de Dios, Javate (1991) 'Struggle against sexual exploitation and prostitution: a Philippine perspective', paper delivered to an International Meeting of Experts, Days Inn State College, Pennsylvania, 8–10 April.

Dworkin, A. (1989) *Pornography: Men Possessing Women*, New York: E.P. Dutton.

Edwards, S. (1981) *Female Sexuality and the Law*, Oxford: Martin Robertson.

Edwards, S. (1984) *Women on Trial*, Manchester: Manchester University Press.

Edwards, S. (1987) 'The kerb-crawling fiasco', *New Law Journal*, 25 Dec.

Edwards, S. (1989) 'Protecting the honour of innocent men', in C. Dunhill (ed.) *The Boys in Blue*, London: Virago.

Edwards, S. (1991a) 'Prostitution: whose problem', Report for the Safer Cities Project, Wolverhampton.

Edwards, S. (1991b) 'The law on the kerb', *Guardian* 4 Oct.

Edwards, S. (1993a) 'Selling the body, keeping the soul', in D. Morgan and S. Scott (eds) *Body Matters*, Falmer Press.

Edwards, S. (1993b) 'Prostitution England and Wales', in Nanette J. Davis (ed.) *Prostitution: an International Handbook on Trends Problems and Policies*, Westport, CT: Greenwood Press.

Edwards, S. and Armstrong, G. (1988) 'Policing prostitution: a profile of the SOS', *Police Journal* July–Sept.: 209–19.

Engels, F. (1986) *The Origin of the Family Private Property and the State*, London: Penguin.

Finstad, L. and Hoigard, C. (1993) 'Norway' [Prostitution in], N.J. Davis (ed.) *Prostitution: An International Handbook on Trends Problems and Policies*, Westport, CT: Greenwood Press.

Giobbe Evelina (1990) 'Confronting the liberal lies about prostitution', in D. Leidholdt and J. Raymond (eds) *The Sexual Liberals and the Attack on Feminism*, Oxford: Pergamon.

Gorham, D. (1978) 'A maiden tribute of modern Babylon re-examined: child prostitution and the idea of childhood in late Victorian England', *Victorian Studies* 21: 353–425.

Jaget, C. (ed.) (1980) *Prostitutes Our Life*, Bristol: Falling Wall Press.

Kollontai, A. (1978) 'Prostitution and ways of fighting it', in *Sexual Relations and the Class Struggle*, London: Allison Busby.

MacKinnon, C. (1982) 'Feminism, Marxism, method and the state: towards a feminist jurisprudence', *Signs: Journal of Women in Culture and Society* 7 (3): 515–44. Reprinted in P.B. Bart and E.G. Moran (1993) *Violence Against Women*, pp. 201–28, Beverly Hills and London: Sage.

Matsui, Y. (1984) 'Why I oppose Kitsaeng', in K. Barry, C. Bunch and S. Castley, *International Feminism: Networking Against Female Sexual Slavery*, New York: International Women's Tribune Center Inc.

McLeod, E. (1982) *Women Working Prostitution Now*, London: Croom Helm.

Meese, E. (1986) *Attorney General's Report on Pornography and Prostitution*, Washington, DC: US Dept of Justice.

Millet, K. (1973) *The Prostitution Papers*, London: Paladin.

Miralao, V. Carlos, C. and Santos, A. (1990) *Women Entertainers in Angeles and Olongopo in the Philippines*, Quezon City, Philippines: Women's Educational Development, Productivity and Research Organisation/Katipuinan ng Kababaihan para sa Kalayaan.

Ohse, U. (1984) *Forced Prostitution and Traffic in Women*, West Germany Human Rights Group.

Pateman, C. (1989) *The Sexual Contract*, Cambridge: Polity Press.

Pheterson, G. (1989) *A Vindication of the Rights of Whores*, Seattle: Seal Press.

Roberts, N. (1986) *The Front Line*, London: Grafton.

Rook, P. and Ward, R. (1990) *Sexual Offences*, The Criminal Law Library, London: Waterlow Publishers/Pergamon Press.

United Nations (1988) *Human Rights A Compilation of International Instruments*, New York: United Nations.

Walkowitz, J. (1977) 'The making of an outcast group: prostitutes and working women in nineteenth-century Plymouth and Southampton', in M. Vicinus (ed.) *A Widening Sphere*, pp. 72–93, London: Methuen.

Wolfenden Committee (1957) *Report on Homosexuality and Prostitution*, Cmnd 24722, London: HMSO.

4 CAMPAIGNING FOR LEGAL CHANGE

Jaget, Claude (ed.) (1980) *Prostitutes – Our Life*, Bristol: Falling Wall Press.

James, Selma (1980) 'Prostitute women and unemployment', speech given at the Institute of Contemporary Arts, 4 December.

James, Selma (1984) 'Hookers in the House of the Lord', in Joy Holland (ed.) *Feminist Action*, London: Battle Axe Books. (Orig. 1983.)

Lopez-Jones, Nina (ed.) (1992) *Prostitute Women and AIDS: Resisting the Virus of Repression*, 2nd edn, London: Crossroads Books.

Network (1983) News from the English Collective of Prostitutes 1 (July).
Power of Women Collective (1975) 'For Prostitutes and Against Prostitution' (leaflet).
RCN (1993) 'Women and men who prostitute', Policy Recommendations, London: Royal College of Nursing.

5 CONSPICUOUS AND INCONSPICUOUS SEX WORK

Adler, F. (1975) *Sisters in Crime: The Rise of the New Female Criminal*, New York: McGraw-Hill.
'Barbara' (1993) 'It's a pleasure doing business with you', *Social Text* 37: 11–22.
Bell, L. (ed.) (1985) *Good Girls/Bad Girls: Sex Trade Workers and Feminists Face to Face*, Toronto, Ontario: The Women's Press.
Boyle, S. (1994) *Working Girls and their Men: Male Sexual Desires and Fantasies Revealed by the Women Paid to Satisfy Them*, London: Smith Gryphon Ltd.
Brittan, A. (1989) *Masculinity and Power*, Oxford: Blackwell.
French, D. (1988) *Working: My Life as a Prostitute*, London: Gollancz.
Giddens, A. (1992) *The Transformation of Intimacy: Sexuality, Love and Eroticism in Modern Society*, Cambridge: Polity Press.
Goffman, E. (1968) *Stigma: The Management of Spoiled Identity*, Harmondsworth: Penguin.
Green, S., Goldberg, D., Christie, P., Frischer, M., Thomson, A., Carr, S. and Taylor, A. (1993) 'Female streetworker-prostitutes in Glasgow: a descriptive study of their lifestyle', *AIDS Care* 5: 321–35.
Hoigard, C. and Finstad, L. (1992) *Backstreets: Prostitution, Money and Love*, Cambridge: Polity Press.
Jaget, C. (ed.) (1980) *Prostitutes: Our Life*, Bristol: Falling Wall Press.
Jarvinen, M. (1993) *Of Vice and Women: Shades of Prostitution*, Scandinavian Studies in Criminology Vol. 13, Oslo: Scandinavian University Press.
'Jasmin' (1993) 'Prostitution is work', *Social Text* 37: 33–7.
McCall, G. and Simmons, J. (1966) *Identities and Interactions: An Examination of Human Associations in Everyday Life*, New York: Free Press.
McCrae, D. (1992) *Nothing Personal: The Business of Sex*, Edinburgh: Mainstream Publishing.
McLeod, E. (1982) *Women Working: Prostitution Now*, London: Croom Helm.
Morgan, M. (1988) 'Dominating the crisis', in I. Reider and P. Ruppelt (eds) *Matters of Life and Death: Women Speak about AIDS*, London: Virago.
Naffine, N. (1987) *Female Crime: The Construction of Women in Criminology*, London: Allen & Unwin.
Perkins, R. and Bennett, G. (1985) *Being a Prostitute: Prostitute Women and Prostitute Men*, Sydney: Allen & Unwin.

Pheterson, G. (1993) 'The whore stigma: female dishonour and male unworthiness', *Social Text* 37: 39–64.

Scambler, G. and Scambler, A. (1995) *Health Issues for Women and Men Sex Workers in London: Final Report*, London: King's Fund.

Scambler, G., Peswani, R., Renton, A. and Scambler, A. (1990) 'Women prostitutes in the AIDS era', *Sociology of Health and Illness* 12: 260–73.

Silver, R. (1993) *The Girl in Scarlet Heels*, London: Century.

Stein, M. (1974) *Lovers, Friends, Slaves . . .*, New York: Berkley Medallion.

Taylor, A. (1991) *Prostitution: What s Love Got to do With It?* London: Macdonald.

Ward, H., Day, S., Mezzone, J., Dunlop, L., Donegan, C., Farrar, S., Whitaker, L., Harris, J. and Miller, D. (1993) 'Prostitution and the risk of HIV: female prostitutes in London', *British Medical Journal* 307: 356–8.

Wellings, K., Field, J., Johnson, A. and Wadsworth, J. (1994) *Sexual Behaviour in Britain: The National Survey of Sexual Attitudes and Lifestyles*, London: Penguin.

Winick, C. (1962) 'Prostitutes' clients' perception of the prostitutes and themselves', *International Journal of Social Psychiatry* 8: 289–97.

6 BOYFRIENDS, 'PIMPS' AND CLIENTS

Armstrong, E.G. (1983) 'Pondering pandering' *Deviant Behaviour* 4 (2): 203–17.

Barry, K. (1995) *Prostitution of Sexuality*, New York, London: New York University Press.

Bourgois, P. and Dunlap, E. (1993) 'Exorcising sex-for-crack: an ethnographic perspective in Harlem', in M.S. Ratner (ed.) *Crack as Pimp: An Ethnographic Investigation of Sex-for-crack Exchanges*, pp. 97–132, New York: Lexington.

Boyle, S. (1994) '*Working Girls and Their Men: Candid Investigation of Prostitution in Britain*, London: Smith Gryphon Ltd.

Chetwynd, J. and Plumridge, E. (1994) 'Knowledge, attitudes and activities of male clients of female sex workers: risk factors for HIV', *New Zealand Medical Journal* 107 (985): 351–3.

Day, S. and Ward, H. (1988) 'Prostitute women and public health', *British Medical Journal* 297: 1585.

Day, S. and Ward, H. (1990) 'The Praed Street project: a cohort of prostitute women in London', in M. Plant (ed.) *AIDS, Drugs and Prostitution*, London: Routledge.

Dorfman, L., Derish, P. and Cohen, J. (1992) '"Hey Girlfriend": an evaluation of AIDS prevention among women in the sex industry', *Health Education Quarterly* 19 (1): 25–40.

Fagan, J. (1994) 'Women and drugs revisited: female participation in the cocaine economy', *Journal of Drug Issues* 24 (2): 179–225.

Faugier, J. (1994) 'Bad women and good customers. Scapegoating, female prostitution and HIV', pp. 50–64 in C. Webb (ed.) *Living Sexuality: Issues for Nursing and Health*, London: Scutari Press.

Faugier, J. (1996) 'Looking for business: a descriptive study of drug using female prostitutes, their clients and their health care needs', PhD thesis, Manchester University.

Faugier, J. and Cranfield, S. (1995) 'Reaching male clients of female prostitutes – the challenge for HIV prevention', *AIDS Cave – Psychological and Socio-medical Aspects of AIDS/HIV* 7 (1): 21–32.

Feldman, H.W., Espada, F., Penn, S. and Bryd, S. (1993) 'Street status and the sex-for-crack scene in San Francisco', in M.S. Ratner (ed.): *Crack as Pimp: An Ethnographic Investigation of Sex-for-crack Exchanges*, pp. 133–58, New York: Lexington.

Feucht, T.E. (1993) 'Prostitutes on crack cocaine: addiction, utility, and marketplace economics', *Deviant Behavior* 14 (2): 91–108.

French, J. (1993) 'Pipe dreams: crack and the life in Philadelphia and Newark', in M.S. Ratner (ed.) *Crack as Pimp: An Ethnographic Investigation of Sex-for-crack Exchanges*, New York: Lexington.

Giobbe, E. (1987) 'WHISPER Oral History Project', Minneapolis, Minnesota.

Girtler, R. (1984) 'Die Prostituierte und ihre Kunden' (The prostitute and her clients), *Kolner Zeitschrift fur Soziologie und Sozialpsychologie* 36 (2): 323–41.

Goldstein, P.J. (1979) *Prostitution and Drugs*, New York: Lexington.

Goldstein, P.J., Ouellet, L.J. and Fendrich, M. (1992) 'From bag brides to skeezers: a historical perspective on sex-for-drugs behavior', *Journal of Psychoactive Drugs* 24 (4): 349–61.

Hardesty, L. and Greif, D.S.W. (1994) 'Common themes in a group for female IV drug users who are HIV positive', *Journal of Psychoactive Drugs* 26 (3): 289–93.

Holland, J., Ramazanoglu, C., Scott, S. *et al.* (1990) 'Sex gender and power, young women's sexuality in the shadow of AIDS', *Sociology of Health and Illness* 12: 336–50.

Inciardi, J.A. Lockwood, D. and Pottieger, A.E. (1993) *Women and Crack-cocaine*, New York: Macmillan.

Jarvinen, M. (1993) *Of Vice and Women: Shades of Prostitution*, Scandinavian Studies in Criminology Vol. 13, Oslo: Scandinavian University Press.

Jolin, A. (1994) 'On the back of working prostitutes: feminist theory and prostitution policy', *Crime and Delinquency* 40: 69–83.

Klee, H., Faugier, J.M. and Hayes, C. (1990) 'Sexual partners of injecting drug users: the risk of HIV infection', *British Journal of Addiction* 85 (3): 413–18.

Leonard, T.L. (1990) 'Male clients of female street prostitutes: unseen partners in sexual disease transmission', *Medical Anthropology Quarterly*, 4 (1): 41–55.

McKeganey, N.P. and Barnard, M.A. (1992a) *AIDS, Drugs and Sexual Risk*, Buckingham: Open University Press.

McKeganey, N.P. and Barnard, M.A. (1992b) 'Selling sex: female street prostitution and HIV risk behaviour in Glasgow', *AIDS Care* 4 (4): 395–407.

McKeganey, N.P., Barnard, M.A., Bloor, M.J. and Leyland, A.C. (1990)

'Injecting drug use and female street-working in Glasgow', *AIDS* 1: 1153–5.

McKeganey, M., Barnard, N. and Leyland, A. (1993) 'Risk behaviours among male clients of female prostitutes', *British Medical Journal* 307: 361–2.

Miller, J. (1995) 'Gender and power on the streets: street prostitution in the era of crack cocaine', *Journal of Contemporary Ethnography* 23: 427–52.

Milner, Christina and Milner, Richard (1972) *Black Players*, Boston: Little, Brown.

Morgan Thomas, R. (1990) 'AIDS risks, alcohol, drugs and the sex industry: a Scottish study', in M. Plant (ed.) *AIDS, Drugs and Prostitution*, London: Routledge.

New York State (1989) *Uniform Crime Report*, New York.

Nichols, P. (1989) *Mobilizing Against AIDS*, Cambridge, MA: Harvard University Press.

Ouellet, L.J., Wiebel, W.W., Jimenez, A.D. and Johnson, W.A. (1993) 'Crack cocaine and the transformation of prostitution in three Chicago neighborhoods'. in M.S. Ratner (ed.) '*Crack as Pimp: An Ethnographic Investigation of Sex-for-crack Exchanges*, New York: Lexington.

Pateman, C. (1988) *The Sexual Contract*, Cambridge: Polity Press.

Perry, L. (1991) 'Women and drug use: an unfeminine dependency', London: Institute for Drug Dependence.

Ratner, M.S. (ed.) (1993) '*Crack as Pimp: An Ethnographic Investigation of Sex-for-crack Exchanges*, New York: Lexington.

Rio, L. (1991) 'Psychological and sociological research and the decriminalization or legalization of prostitution', *Archives of Sexual Behavior* 20 (2): 205–18.

Rosenbaum, W. (1981) *Women on heroin*, New Brunswick, NJ: Rutgers University Press.

Sacks, V. (1996) 'Women and AIDS: an analysis of media misrepresentations', *Social Science and Medicine* 42 (1): 59–73.

Sherr, L. and Hedge, B. (1990) 'The impact of using written leaflets as a counselling alternative in mass ante-natal screening', *AIDS Care* 2 (3): 235–47.

Silbert, M.H. and Pines, A.M. (1982) 'Victimization of street prostitutes', *Victimology* 7 (1–4): 122–33.

Slim, Iceberg (1969) *Pimp: The Story of My Life*, Los Angeles: Holloway.

Stephens, R.C. (1991) *The Street Addict Role: A Theory of Heroin Addiction*, Buffalo: SUNY Press.

Walkowitz, J. (1980) *Prostitution and the Victorian City: Women, Class and the State*, Cambridge: Cambridge University Press.

Williams, T. (1992) *Crackhouse*, Reading, MA: Addison-Wesley.

7 HEALTH CARE AND REGULATION

Allen, J. (1984) 'The making of a prostitute proletariat in early 20th-century New South Wales', in K. Daniels (ed.) *So Much Hard Work*, Sydney: Fontana/Collins.

Barton, S.E., Taylor-Robinson, D. and Harris, J.R.W. (1987) 'Female prostitutes and sexually transmitted diseases', *British Journal of Hospital Medicine* 7: 34–45.

Brunham, R.C. (1991) 'The concept of cores and its relevance to the epidemiology and control of sexually transmitted diseases', *Sexually Transmitted Diseases* 18 (2): 67–71.

Casey, M., Day, S., Ward, H. and Ziersch, A. (1995) *Sexual Health Services for Prostitutes in the UK*. Published by Europap (UK).

Centres for Disease Control (1987) 'Antibody to human immunodeficiency virus in female prostitutes', *MMWR* 36: 157–61.

Day, S. (1988) 'Prostitute women and AIDS: Anthropology', *AIDS*, 2 421–8.

Day S., Ward H. and Harris, J.R.W. (1988) 'Prostitute women and public health', *British Medical Journal* 297: 1585.

Delgado, M. (1992) 'Police issue AIDS alert over King's Cross prostitutes', *Evening Standard* 17 March.

Elias, J.E. and Heise, L. (1994) 'Challenges for the development of female-controlled vaginal microbicides', *AIDS* 8: 1–9.

EUROPAP (1995) *Final Report to the European Commission*, February.

European Working Group on HIV Infection in Female Prostitutes (1993) HIV infection in European female sex workers: epidemiological link with use of petroleum-based lubricants', *AIDS* 7: 401–8.

Krogsgard, K., Gluud, C., Pederson, C. *et al.* (1986) 'Widespread use of condoms and low prevalence of sexually transmitted diseases in Danish non-drug addicted prostitutes', *British Medical Journal* 293: 1473–7.

McKeganey, N., Barnard, M., Leyland, A. *et al.* (1992) 'Female street-working prostitution and HIV infection in Glasgow', *British Medical Journal* 305: 801–4.

Neequaya A.R., Neequaya, J., Mingle, J.A. *et al.* (1986) 'Preponderance of females with AIDS in Ghana', *Lancet* ii: 978.

Overs, C. (1994) 'Sex work, HIV and the state: an interview with Nel Druce', *Feminist Review* 48: 114–21.

Perkins, R. and Bennett, G. (1985) *Being a Prostitute*, Sydney: George Allen & Unwin.

Piot, P., Plummer, F.A. and Rey, M.A. *et al.* (1987) 'Retrospective sero-epidemiology of AIDS virus infection in Nairobi populations', *Journal of Infectious Disease* 155: 1108–12.

Plummer, F.A., Nagelkerke, N.J.D., Moses, S., Ndinya-Achola, J.O., Bwayo, J. and Ngugi, E. (1991) 'The importance of core groups in the epidemiology and control of HIV-1 infection', *AIDS* 5 (suppl.): S169–76.

Queen, H.F., Ward, H., Smith, C. and Woodroffe, C. (1991) 'Potential for better co-ordination of women's health services', *Genitourinary Medicine* 67: 215–19.

Smith, G.L. and Smith, K.F. (1987) 'Lack of HIV infection and condom use in licensed prostitutes', *Lancet*, ii: 1392.

Sunday Express (1992) 'Met has mugshots of hookers with AIDS', 29 March.

Thomas, R.M., Plant, M.A., Plant, M.L. and Sales, J. (1990) 'Risk of HIV infection among clients of the sex industry in Scotland', *British Medical Journal* 301: 525.

van den Hoek, J.A. and van Haastrecht, H.J.A. (1988) 'Prevalence and risk factors for HIV infection among drug users and drug using prostitutes in Amsterdam', *AIDS* 2: 55–60.

Van de Perre, P. (1985) 'Female prostitutes: a risk group for infection with human T-cell lymphotropic virus type III', *Lancet* ii: 524.

Walkowitz, J. (1980) *Prostitution and Victorian Society: women, class and the state*, Cambridge: Cambridge University Press.

Ward, H. and Day, S. (1991) 'Prostitution', in J.R.W. Harris and S. Forster (eds) *Recent Advances in STD and AIDS – 4*, Edinburgh: Churchill Livingstone.

Ward, H. and Day, S.E. (1992) 'Recording HIV status on police computers', *British Medical Journal* 304: 1635–6.

Ward, H., Day, S., Mezzone, J., Dunlop, L., Donegan, C., Farrar, S., Whitaker, L., Harris, J.R.W., and Miller, D.L. (1993) Prostitution and risk of HIV: female prostitutes in London, *British Medical Journal* 307: 356–8.

Ward, H., de la Court, A. and Kitchen, V. (in press) 'Nonoxynol-9 in lubricated condoms – results of a pilot study in prostitute women', *Sexually Transmitted Diseases*.

Weir, S.S., Roddy, R.E., Zekeng, L. and Feldblum, P.J. (1995) 'Nonoxynol-9 use, genital ulcers, and HIV infection in a cohort of sex workers', *Genitourinary Medicine* 71: 78–81.

Woolley, P.D., Bowman, C.A. and Kinghorn, G.R. (1988) 'Prostitution in Sheffield: differences between prostitutes', *Genitourinary Medicine* 64: 391–3.

8 ALCOHOL, DRUGS AND SOCIAL MILIEU

Anderson, K. and Plant, M.A. (in press) 'Abstaining and carousing: substance use amongst adolescents in the Western Isles', *Drug and Alcohol Dependence*.

Bloor, M., Leyland, A., Barnard, M. and McKeganey, N. (1991) 'Estimating hidden populations: a new method of calculating the prevalence of drug-injecting and non-injecting female street prostitution', *British Journal of Addiction* 86: 1477–83.

Bush, P. J. (1980) *Drugs, Alcohol and Sex*, New York: Marek.

Carr, S.T., Green, S.T., Goldberg, D., Cameron, S., Gruer, L., Frischer, M., Mackie, T. and Follett, E. (1992) 'HIV prevalence amongst female street prostitutes attending a health care drop-in centre in Glasgow', (letter) *AIDS*, 6: 1553–4.

Cavan, S. (1966) *Liquor License: An Ethnography of Bar Behavior*, Chicago: Aldine.

Coles, R. and Stokes, G. (1985) *Sex and the American Teenager*, New York: Harper & Row.

Davies, J.B. and Stacey, B. (1972) *Teenagers and Alcohol*, London, HMSO.

De Graaf, R., Vanwesenbeeck, I., van Zessen, G., Straver, C.J. and Visser, J.H. (1994) 'Male prostitutes and safe sex: different settings, different risks', *AIDS Care* 6: 277–88.

De Graaf, R., Vanwesenbeeck, G., van Zessen, G., Straver, C.J. and Visser, J.H. (1995) 'Alcohol and drug use in heterosexual and homosexual prostitution and its relation to protection behaviour', *AIDS Care* 7: 35–47.

Edlin, B.R., Irwin, K.L., Ludwig, D.D., McCoy, H.V., Serrano, Y., Word, C., Bowser, B.P., Faruque, S., McCoy, C.B., Schilling, R.F., Holmberg, S.D. and the Multicentre Crack Cocaine and HIV Infection Study Team (1992) 'High risk sex behavior among young street recruited crack cocaine smokers in three American cities: an interim report', *Journal of Psychoactive Drugs*, 24: 363–71.

Elifson, K.W., Boles, J. and Sweat, M. (1993) 'Risk factors associated with HIV infection among male prostitutes', *American Journal of Public Health* 83: 79–83.

Farley, T.A., Hadler, J.L. and Gunn, R.A. (1990) 'The syphilis epidemic in Connecticut: relationship to drug use and prostitution', *Sexually Transmitted Diseases* Oct.–Dec.: 163–8.

Fossey, E. (1994) *Growing Up with Alcohol*, London: Tavistock/Routledge.

Foster, K., Wilmot, A. and Dobbs, J. (1990) *General Household Survey 1988*, London: HMSO.

Gill, J. (1994) 'Alcohol problems in employment: epidemiology and responses', *Alcohol and Alcoholism* 29: 233–48.

Goldberg, D., Green, S.T., Taylor, A., Frischer, M. and McKeganey, N. (1994) 'Comparison of four survey methods designed to estimate the prevalence of HIV among female prostitutes who inject drugs', *International Journal of STD and AIDS* 5: 186–8.

Gossop, M., Griffiths, P., Powis, B. and Strang, J. (1993) 'Severity of heroin dependence and HIV risk, 1: sexual behaviour', AIDS *Care* 5 149–57.

Gossop, M., Powis, B., Griffiths, P. and Strang, J. (1994) 'Sexual behaviour and its relationship to drug-taking among prostitutes in south London', *Addiction* 89: 961–70.

Green, S.T., Taylor, A., Fischer, M. and Goldberg, D.J. (1993) 'Frontloading (halfing) among drug injectors as a continuing risk behaviour for HIV transmission', *Addiction* 88: 1581–2.

Home Office (1995a) *Statistics of Drug Addicts Notified to the Home Office, United Kingdom 1994*, London: Home Office.

Home Office (1995b) *Statistics of Drug Seizures and Offenders Dealt With, United Kingdom, 1993*, London: Home Office.

Hutcheson, G.D., Henderson, M. and Davies, J.B. (1995) *Alcohol in the Workplace*, Research Series No. 59, London: Department of Employment.

Leigh, B.C. and Stall, R. (1993) 'Substance use and risky sexual behaviour', *Journal of Sex Research* 27: 199–213.

Loretto, W. (1994) 'Youthful drinking in Northern Ireland and Scotland: preliminary results from a comparative study', *Drugs: Education, Prevention and Policy* 1: 143–52.

McDonald, M. (ed.) (1995) *Gender, Drink and Drugs*, Oxford: Berg.

McKeganey, N. and Barnard, M. (1992) *AIDS, Drugs and Sexual Risk*, Milton Keynes: Open University Press.

McKeganey, N., Barnard, M., Bloor, M. and Leyland, A. (1990) 'Injecting drug use and female street working prostitutes in Glasgow', *AIDS* 4: 1153–5.

McKeganey, N., Barnard, M., Leyland, A., Coote, I. and Follet, E. (1992) 'Female streetworking prostitution and HIV infection in Glasgow', *British Medical Journal* 305: 801–4.

Matthews L. (1990) 'Outreach work with female prostitutes in Liverpool', in M.A. Plant (ed.) *AIDS, Drugs and Prostitution*, pp. 76–87, London: Tavistock/Routledge.

May, C. (1992) 'A burning issue? Adolescent alcohol use in Britain 1970–1991', *Alcohol and Alcoholism* 27: 109–15.

Miller, P., Plant, M.L., Plant, M.A. and Duffy, J. (1995) 'Alcohol, tobacco, illicit drugs and sex: an analysis of risky behaviours among young adults', *International Journal of the Addictions* 30: 239–58.

Morgan Thomas, R. (1990) 'AIDS risks, alcohol drugs and the sex industry; a Scottish study', in M.A. Plant (ed.) *AIDS, Drugs and Prostitution*, pp. 88–108, London: Tavistock/Routledge.

Morgan Thomas, R (1995) Personal communication.

Morgan Thomas, R., Plant, M.A., Plant, M.L. and Sales, D.I. (1989) 'Risk of AIDS among workers in the "sex industry": some initial results from a Scottish study', *British Medical Journal* 299: 148–9.

Morgan Thomas, R., Plant, M.A. and Plant, M.L. (1990a) 'Alcohol, AIDS risks and sex industry clients: results from a Scottish study', *Drug and Alcohol Dependence* 26: 265–9.

Morgan Thomas, R., Plant, M.A., Plant, M.L. and Sales, J. (1990b) 'Risk of HIV infection among clients of the sex industry in Scotland', *British Medical Journal*, 301: 525.

Morrison, C.L., Ruben, S. and Wakefield, D. (1994) 'Female street prostitution in Liverpool' (letter), *AIDS* 8: 1194–5.

Morrison, C.L., McGee, A. and Ruben, S.M. (1995) 'Alcohol and drug misuse in prostitutes' (letter), *Addiction* 90: 292–3.

Parker, H., Measham, F. and Aldridge, J. (1995) *Drugs Futures: Changing Patterns of Drug Use Amongst English Youth*, London: Institute for the Study of Drug Dependence.

Philpot, C.R., Harcourt, C. and Edwards, J.M. (1989) 'Drug use by Sydney prostitutes', *British Journal of Addiction* 84: 499–505.

Plant, M.A. (1979) *Drinking Careers*, London: Tavistock.

Plant, M.A. (ed.) (1990) *AIDS, Drugs and Prostitution*, London: Tavistock/Routledge.

Plant, M.A. (1993) 'Alcohol, AIDS and sex', in: L. Sherr (ed.) *Heterosexual AIDS*, pp. 223–40, Switzerland: Harwood.

Plant, M.A. (1996) 'Contemporary research – alcohol, drugs, HIV/AIDS and risk taking', *Journal of Substance Misuse for Nursing, Health and Social Care* 1: 32–7.

Plant, M.A. and Foster, J. (1991) 'Teenagers and alcohol: results of a Scottish national survey', *Drug and Alcohol Dependence* 28: 203–10.

Plant, M.A., Bagnall, G., Foster, J. and Sales, J. (1990) 'Young people and drinking: results of an English national survey', *Alcohol and Alcoholism* 25: 685–90.

Plant, M.A. and Plant, M.L. (1992) *Risk Takers: Alcohol, Drugs, Sex and Youth*, London: Tavistock/Routledge.

Plant, M.L. (1990) *Women and Alcohol*, Copenhagen: World Health Organization.

Plant, M.L., Plant, M.A. and Morgan Thomas, R. (1990) 'Alcohol, AIDS risks and commercial sex: some preliminary results from a Scottish study', *Drug and Alcohol Dependence* 25: 51–55.

Rhodes, T., Donoghue., M., Hunter, G. and Stimson, G.V. (1994) 'HIV prevalence no higher among female drug injectors also involved in prostitution', *AIDS Care* 6: 269–76.

Ridlon, F.V. (1988) *Fallen Angel: The Status Insularity of the Female Alcoholic*, London: Bucknell University Press.

Room, R. and Collins, G. (eds) (1983) *Alcohol and Disinhibition: Nature and Meaning of the Link*, Research Monograph No. 12, Rockville, Maryland: National Institute on Alcohol Abuse and Alcoholism.

Soloman, D. and Andrews, G. (eds) (1973) *Drugs and Sexuality*, St Albans: Panther.

Stall, R., McKusick, and Wiley, J. (1986) 'Alcohol and drug use during sexual activity and compliance with safe sex guidelines for AIDS: the AIDS Behavioral Research Project', *Health Education Quarterly* 13: 359–71.

Strang, J. and Stimson, G.V. (1990) *AIDS and Drug Misuse*, London: Tavistock/Routledge.

Taylor, A., Frischer, M., McKeganey, N., Goldberg, D., Green, S. and Platt, S. (1993) 'HIV risk behaviours among female prostitute drug injectors in Glasgow', *Addiction* 88: 1561–4.

van der Hoek, J.A.R., van der Linden, M.M.D. and Coutinho, R.A. (1990) 'Increase of infectious syphilis among heterosexuals in Amsterdam: its relationship to drug use and prostitution', *Genitourinary Medicine* 66: 31–21.

van den Hoek, J.A.R., van Haastrecht, H.J.A. and Coutinho, R.A. (1991) 'Homosexual prostitution among male drug users and its risk for HIV infection', *Genitourinary Medicine* 67: 303–6.

Weatherburn, P. (1994) personal communication.

World Health Organization (1994) *Alcohol and HIV/AIDS*, Copenhagen: World Health Organization Regional Office for Europe.

AFTERWORD: RETHINKING PROSTITUTION

Altink, S. (1995) *Stolen Lives: Trading Women into Sex and Slavery*, London: Scarlet Press.

Carroll, N. and Scambler, G. (1992) 'Public attitude towards women sex workers against the background of the AIDS epidemic', unpublished manuscript.

Ericsson, L. (1980) 'Charges against prostitution: an attempt at a philosophical assessment', *Ethics 90*: 335–66.

Lemert, E. (1967) *Human Deviance, Social Problems and Social Control*, New York: Prentice-Hall.

Matthews, R. (1986) 'Beyond Wolfenden? Prostitution, politics and the law', in R. Matthews and J. Young (eds) *Confronting Crime*, London: Sage.

Pateman, C. (1983) 'Defending prostitution: charges against Ericsson', *Ethics*, 93: 561–5.

Pheterson, G. (ed.) (1989) *A Vindication of the Rights of Whores*, Seattle: Free Press.

Primoratz, I. (1993) 'What's wrong with prostitution?' *Philosophy* 68: 159–82.

Roberts, N. (1992) *Whores in History: Prostitution in Western Society*, London: HarperCollins.

Scambler, G. and Scambler, A. (1994) 'Health promotion, the sex industry and the challenge of change', *Critical Public Health* 5: 30–35.

Scambler, G. and Scambler, A. (1995) 'Social change and health promotion among women sex workers in London', *Health Promotion International* 10: 17–24.

Scambler, G., Peswani, R., Renton, A. and Scambler, A. (1990) 'Women prostitutes in the AIDS era', *Sociology of Health and Illness* 12: 260–73.

Shrage, L. (1989) 'Should feminists oppose prostitution?' *Ethics* 99: 347–61.

Shrage, L. (1994) *Moral Dilemmas of Feminism: Prostitution, Adultery and Abortion*, London: Routledge.

Wilson, E. (1983) *What is to be Done about Violence against Women?* Harmondsworth: Penguin.

Index